D1084938

STROKE

**Recent Titles in the
Biographies of Disease Series**

Parkinson's Disease
Nutan Sharma

Depression
Blaise A. Aguirre

Diabetes
Andrew Galmer

STROKE

Jonathan A. Edlow

Biographies of Disease
Julie K. Silver, M.D., Series Editor

GREENWOOD PRESS
Westport, Connecticut • London

Library of Congress Cataloging-in-Publication Data

Edlow, Jonathan A.
 Stroke / Jonathan A. Edlow.
  p. ; cm.—(Biographies of disease, ISSN 1940-445X)
 Includes bibliographical references and index.
 ISBN 978-0-313-34241-7 (alk. paper)
 1. Cerebrovascular disease. I. Title. II. Series.
 [DNLM: 1. Stroke. WL 355 E23s 2008]
 RC388.5.E323 2008
 616.8′1—dc22   2008004527

British Library Cataloguing in Publication Data is available.

Library of Congress Catalog Card Number: 2008004527
ISBN: 978-0-313-34241-7
ISSN: 1940-445X

First published in 2008

Greenwood Press, 88 Post Road West, Westport, CT 06881
An imprint of Greenwood Publishing Group, Inc.
www.greenwood.com

Printed in the United States of America

The paper used in this book complies with the
Permanent Paper Standard issued by the National
Information Standards Organization (Z39.48–1984).

10 9 8 7 6 5 4 3 2 1

Contents

Series Foreword

E very killer has a story to tell, and so it is with diseases as well: about how it started long ago and began to take the lives of its innocent victims, about the way it hurts us, and about how we are trying to stop it. In this *Biographies of Disease* series, the authors tell the stories of the diseases that we have come to know and fear.

The stories of these killers have all of the components that make for great literature. There is incredible drama played out in real-life scenes from the past, present, and future. You'll read about how men and women of science stumbled trying to save the lives of those they aimed to protect. Turn the pages and you'll also learn about the amazing success of those who fought the killer and won, saving thousands of lives in the process.

If you don't want to be a health professional or research scientist now, when you finish this book you may think differently. The men and women in this book are heroes who often risked their own lives to save ours. This is the biography of a killer, but it is also the story of real people who made incredible sacrifices to stop it in its tracks.

Julie K. Silver, M.D.
Assistant Professor, Harvard Medical School
Department of Physical Medicine and Rehabilitation

Preface

When I was in high school, my grandfather had a severe stroke. He was a diabetic, and, in those days, the late 1960s, doctors did not have their patients control their blood sugars very closely. Diabetes was, and as the reader will see still is, an important risk factor for stroke. His stroke was a scary thing for the family. He was hospitalized in a medium-sized hospital in downtown Baltimore, close to where he worked but far from where we lived. I remember my cousin Jay, a medical student at the time, drove some of the family to the hospital.

At his bedside, although I knew no more about stroke than the average high school student, I can recall three things. The first is that my grandfather could not speak, not even a single word. The second is that he could not move the right side of his body at all, but, when I stood on his left, he would squeeze my hand, strongly, with his left hand. I don't know why I remember that, but I do. The third memory is how devastating the stroke was for the family. It was frightening to have a loved one who is normal one minute and literally paralyzed and mute the next.

I didn't know that I was going to become a doctor, nor was this any defining moment of my adolescence. In fact, I haven't thought of it for many years, but the experience obviously left a mark. I think that the reason that the memory comes to mind as I write this preface is that the real impact on society is the human impact that stroke imparts onto its victims and their families.

As a doctor, I see patients with strokes with some frequency and sometimes must remind myself about the human consequences. As a high school student, to whom this book is targeted, I only remember the fear and sorrow. Hopefully, the information in this book will elevate the knowledge about stroke for the reader and create light where there was previously darkness.

Stroke remains a devastating illness, and, despite our improved understanding of risk factors and prevention, it is getting more common, not less. This is mostly because the amount of the population that is elderly is increasing, a function of the "baby boomers" born after World War II coming of "old" age.

This book discusses all aspects of stroke. It starts out by defining exactly what the term means and explaining some of the relevant anatomy so that the reader will understand the various kinds of stroke. Subsequent chapters describe the risk factors and the underlying physiology of stroke, what symptoms patients have, and how doctors diagnose stroke. Various treatments are discussed in some detail. These are chapters that would have been rather sparse a mere twenty years ago because many of the therapies are relatively new.

Later chapters discuss the outcomes of stroke patients and how doctors measure them. Prevention of stroke is also discussed in two chapters, the second of which outlines the very important topic of "TIA" (transient ischemic attack), which is an important component to understand. Last, the book closes with new ideas that are not yet standard medical care, although many of the issues and treatments discussed in this last chapter may become standard in another five years.

In addition, the book contains a few other features, such as a timeline that shows what was known about stroke when; fortunately for those of us alive today, this timeline is very "end-loaded" because much of the practical information we know about stroke has only come to light in recent years. A glossary includes most of the important medical terms that are not widely known.

Last, there are a few people I would like to acknowledge. The first is Dr. Julie Silvers, who first asked me to join this project. Thanks for the invitation! Second, I thank Dr. Anil Shukla, a physician in training who is also a spectacular artist. Anil rendered the line drawings that illustrate various anatomic points. His artwork helps enormously to give shape and meaning to the words on the page. Thank you, Anil. Last, I thank my wife, Pamela, who carefully edited the entire document and helped to translate my sometimes awkward and over-medicalized language into English. Thank you, Pam!

Finally, I dedicate this book to my son, Julian Edlow, a sophomore in college as I write these words. May you always continue to learn and, as your father did, stumble on the subject that makes you happy and keeps your creative juices flowing.

1

Introductory Concepts and Definitions

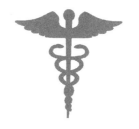

For the New England Patriots football team, the 2004–2005 season was one of their best ever. On Sunday, February 6, 2005, the Patriots won their third Super Bowl in just four years. People were using terms like "sports dynasty" when talking about quarterback Tom Brady and Coach Bill Belichick as if they were unstoppable. A huge part of the team's success was credited to their defense. Tedy Bruschi was the heart of that defense and the captain of the team. At 6'1" and 245 pounds, he was handsome, muscular, and the picture of health, with a strong jaw and an easy smile. Married to his long-time love, Heidi, and building a family, Tedy was considered a great guy, and the fans adored him.

At just thirty-one years old, Tedy was at the peak of his football career, a sport he chose to pursue over wrestling, track, and playing the sax, just a few of the things he excelled in during high school.

After the Super Bowl, Bruschi had been selected to play in the Pro Bowl, an annual event that honors the best in the National Football League. Along with quarterback Tom Brady and a few other teammates, Bruschi joined many of the premier players in the National Football League in this game, which is traditionally held in Hawaii. Even for West Coasters, that means a minimum of a six-hour plane flight, but for a New Englander like Bruschi, the flight was twelve hours long. The game took place on Sunday, February 13, just a week after his stellar performance in the Super Bowl. He played hard in the game, like he does in every game he plays, and then flew home to Massachusetts.

He was home less than two days when, on February 16, he awoke at 4:00 A.M. feeling numb on the left side of his body. According to newspaper accounts, he also had some problems with balance and experienced pain in the back of his neck. Bruschi and Heidi discussed it briefly, and then, concluding that it was just one of those things that he would shake off, they went back to sleep. However, when Tedy Bruschi woke up again at about 10:00 A.M., the odd neurological symptoms were still there. Even then, the football player was not sure whether he needed to see a doctor, but he quickly changed his mind.

"But even then I was saying, 'I don't know if I need to go,'" Bruschi said in a *Boston Globe* interview (MacMullan, September 2, 2005). "I was thinking it was something that could possibly pass. I didn't have a tremendous amount of pain." It wasn't until his five-year-old son, Tedy Jr., scampered into the room that the linebacker realized the severity of his condition. "TJ came in from my left," Bruschi said. "I heard him, but I didn't see him. I didn't see him until he popped up on the right side of my field of vision and said, 'Good morning, Daddy.' That's when I got scared. I told Heidi, 'Call 911.'"

Speaking calmly to the 911 dispatcher, Heidi Bruschi said that her husband was suffering from "blurred vision and numbness on the right side of his body." The dispatcher knew to send help immediately.

Bruschi was rushed by ambulance to Massachusetts General Hospital. Within minutes of hitting the emergency department (ED), a protocol would have been followed. His pulse and blood pressure were taken, and an intravenous line was inserted and hooked up to a cardiac monitor to measure his heart-beat. A doctor would have rapidly determined what his symptoms were and performed a quick physical examination. This would have been followed by a computed tomographic (CT) scan of his brain.

"Within minutes of the CT scan, the doctor came out, put his hand on my shoulder, and said, 'You've had a mild stroke,'" Bruschi recalled. "I said, 'What?' I was in disbelief. It was a total shock to me."

Tedy Bruschi, about as healthy a human specimen as one could imagine, had just had a stroke!

Another famous (and seemingly healthy) person who suffered a stroke is actress Sharon Stone. In September 2001, at the age of 43, the attractive, blonde actress who starred in the blockbuster *Basic Instinct* developed a severe headache, much more intense than the migraines that she sometimes had. On September 29, a number of days after thinking the headache would resolve at home, she was hospitalized. Her CT scan also showed a stroke but a very different kind than Tedy Bruschi's. She had a condition called a subarachnoid hemorrhage: bleeding around the outside of her brain. She underwent two different angiograms, which is an x-ray of the blood vessels, the second of which finally showed the cause: a tear in an artery of the brain.

Bruschi and Stone were fortunate; they both received expert treatment and both returned to the professions they love. Not all stroke patients survive and not all survivors recover to that same extent.

The Greeks and Romans knew almost nothing about stroke. This is best illustrated by the very word that they used to describe the condition: apoplexy. This work in Greek means "struck down by violence," suggesting that some mysterious force from outside of the body is responsible for the symptoms. The specific concept that there was a problem in the brain did not occur until 1658. At that time, Johann Jakob Wepfer, working at the University of Padua in Italy, theorized that a broken brain blood vessel may cause apoplexy. He spent countless hours dissecting brains of patients who had died of stroke, and he found that blocked or ruptured arteries to the brain were the problem. His discovery was not greeted with much enthusiasm, however, because during the Renaissance diseases such as smallpox, plague, and tuberculosis were much more feared than apoplexy.

During the 1700s and 1800s, the anatomy of the brain was worked out in fairly elegant detail, but doctors still did not know much about causes of stroke and certainly had no treatments. As well, during the latter half of the 1800s, doctors began to have a greater appreciation of the interaction between the cerebral blood vessels and stroke. However, it was not until the middle of the past century when more sophisticated research was done about the exact causes of stroke. Despite these brilliant advances, little progress was made on treatment of the devastating condition. It has only been during the past few decades that important advances have been made in stroke treatment and prevention.

By itself, the word "stroke" does not convey very much. When someone has a "heart attack," two things are pretty clear. You at least know what body part is involved, the heart, and there is something about the phrase that conveys a sense of urgency. Similarly, terms like "kidney stone" or "sprained ankle" tell you a little bit about the problem. However, "stroke" does not tell you very much, does it? It certainly does not specify what body part is involved, nor does it convey much information about how serious a problem it is.

However, the word "stroke" does reveal one very important and descriptive element of the word: an abrupt onset. The word "stroke" when used in, say, golf or tennis, conveys an event that happens in an instant, like Tiger Woods's golf swing or Roger Federer's forehand.

In medical jargon, a stroke is the condition in which part of the brain abruptly loses its source of nutrients, oxygen and glucose, that are normally delivered to it by way of the vascular system. Normally, with each beat, the heart pumps blood into its major outflow artery called the aorta. This blood is rich in oxygen as a result of having passed through the lungs. It also carries adequate amounts of glucose, a kind of sugar, to all organs in the body. The brain is the hungriest and is constantly using these two essential ingredients to fuel its tangled factory of nerve cells and their connections. Deprive the brain of this fuel for even a few moments and a person will rapidly lose consciousness.

This is what happens in a common fainting episode. The blood pressure plummets and the brain is deprived of oxygen and glucose. Seconds later, the person will faint. Once they are on the ground in a horizontal position, their blood can circulate more easily. This normally allows a person's blood pressure to rise enough to supply the brain with its normal needs. The person wakes up. This is why it is important when you are helping someone who feels faint or who has fainted to lie them down flat on the ground, but a fainting episode is not the same as a stroke. What is the difference?

The adult human brain is a three-pound gelatinous mass. Although it only represents 2 percent of your body weight, it receives approximately 15 percent of your entire body's blood flow. This gives you an idea of how dependent on oxygen and glucose the brain is. No other organ in the body gets so much blood flow. We have evolved this way for a reason; our brains are the most important structure that has allowed us to distinguish ourselves from other animals. Our brains allow us to adapt to limitless situations, whether it's reacting to a pitched ball that speeds at us from the pitcher's mound or to a dog that has suddenly run out in front of the car, of whether it's creating important, new inventions, simply studying for a math test or learning how to play the saxophone.

Think about what happens in this last example, and let's make it more specific, say, playing the saxophone in a marching band. You may or may not have sheet music in front of you. If you do, you're reading the notes. You're hearing the other members of the band. You're watching the conductor keeping time and you're walking forward all the while.

You "read" the notes on the sheet music using your eyes. Light falls on your retina, which is actually composed of cells from the central nervous system. These photons of light are converted into electronic impulses that are sent through nerve cells through an elaborate pathway in which they are processed into some intelligible meaning. Connections from the optical part of the brain tell another part to make your lungs push a certain amount of air out of your mouth and your lip muscles to have just the right amount of tension to make a certain note. All the while, another part, just a few inches away, is telling your fingers to make the rapid changes so that the notes in the song come out just right.

While all of this is happening, still another area of the brain is controlling your legs, ordering them to march to the beat of the music while the auditory brain is listening to and timing the music. All of these actions are being continually repeated and changing, depending on the notes on the musical score, the directions of the conductor, and the interactions with the other musicians in the band.

It's no wonder that the brain needs its continuous supply of oxygen and glucose, its fuel and power source, when it is performing so many different actions simultaneously. Although this example shows what the brain is capable of in times of relatively high demand, even in more baseline situations, such as reading a book, making a sandwich, or riding a bike, a lot is happening.

When a person has a stroke, one specific area of the brain stops getting enough of these nutrients. Within seconds to minutes, that specific part of the brain stops functioning properly. Like the word implies, this occurs instantly, in the stroke of almost a second.

In fact, one clue that doctors use when trying to determine the cause of a patient's illness is that, if a patient's neurological symptoms developed abruptly, then stroke is a likely diagnosis. The specific part of the brain that loses function depends on which artery is involved. We'll talk more about this in Chapter 3, but for now, let's just say that every function that we have—each of our senses, our ability to move the thumb, or the knee, the sensation of knowing the position of the body, our ability to keep our balance—has its own real estate in the brain.

One person's stroke may involve the part of the brain responsible for seeing objects to the right. Another's may leave them unable to speak, whereas still another may simply lose balance to the extent that they cannot stand upright. So a stroke patient has "focal" symptoms, which is to say that they are attributable to loss of function in one specific part of the brain, that part of the brain that was deprived of its nutrients. This is different from the patient who faints, whose symptoms are attributable to the whole brain temporarily losing blood flow.

The three elements that are common to a stroke are as follows: (1) abrupt onset of focal neurological symptoms, (2) symptoms that can be attributed to losing blood flow in a single artery's territory, and (3) symptoms that last for at least twenty-four hours.

This last element brings up another term that we must understand if we are to understand what a stroke is: transient ischemic attack (TIA). A TIA has both the first two elements of a stroke, but the duration of the symptoms is less. Therefore, a TIA is defined as follows: (1) abrupt onset of focal neurological symptoms, (2) symptoms that can be attributed to losing blood flow in a single artery's territory, and (3) symptoms that last for less than twenty-four hours.

A TIA is like a warning that a full stroke will occur. For decades, physicians have realized that, in the months to years after a TIA, patients had a higher than normal risk of stroke. However, since 2000, doctors have recognized that the risk of a full stroke is higher even in the first days that follow a TIA, as high as 5 percent. That means that, of every twenty persons having a TIA, one will suffer a stroke in the following two days. Some medical studies have even found slightly higher rates of early stroke after TIA.

More recently, physicians who specialize in the care of stroke patients, called stroke neurologists, have begun to debate whether stroke and TIA are really two distinct entities that can be neatly divided based on the duration of the symptoms. We will examine this debate more in later chapters when we learn further about risk factors for stroke, the "anatomy" of strokes, and diagnostic testing. For now, it is enough to know that TIA and stroke are really different presentations of the same problem.

With regard to introductions, there is just one more to be made at the outset. There are different kinds of strokes, and this does not just refer to causes. Doctors make a major distinction between "ischemic" and "hemorrhagic" strokes. An ischemic stroke is one in which a solid blood clot blocks the flow of blood in an artery to the brain. This clot obstructs the flow of blood so that any brain tissue that normally is fed by this artery is deprived of the nutrients (oxygen and glucose) that are normally supplied. A hemorrhagic stroke is one in which a blood vessel bursts and the blood creates pressure on the brain. The common thread in both types is that a problem in a blood vessel in the brain prohibits delivery of the brain's power source, which in turn leads to the death of brain cells. There are several subtypes of both ischemic and hemorrhagic stroke, but we will learn more of these details in later chapters.

That said, this distinction in types of stroke is very important and will need to be reinforced in all subsequent chapters, because risk factors, symptoms, findings on various diagnostic tests, and treatments vary quite a bit between them. In fact, the best treatment for some patients with ischemic stroke would be dangerous in patients with hemorrhagic strokes. This is an important distinction between stroke and, for example, a heart attack. The vast majority of heart attacks are caused by the same pathologic cause: atherosclerosis (blockage) of the coronary (heart) arteries. The pathology and causes (pathophysiology) of stroke are much more varied. Not surprisingly, because there are many kinds of strokes, there are different symptoms and different treatments. This makes stroke research a bit more difficult than, say, research for heart attacks, but again, we will learn more about this later.

Unfortunately, what happened to Tedy Bruschi is not so uncommon, and he is not the only well-known person to have a stroke. Ted Williams, the baseball Hall-of-Famer, had a stroke. Former Miss America Jacquelyn Jeanne Mayer suffered a near-fatal stroke in 1970, at the age of only twenty-eight. Her stroke was more serious than Bruschi's, and she spent seven years in rehabilitation relearning basic activities of daily living, such as the ability to walk and speak. Politicians like Senator Joe Biden, Israeli Prime Minister Ariel Sharon, and historic figures such as Winston Churchill, Franklin Roosevelt, and Josef Stalin all suffered strokes. So did actors Kirk Douglas, Robert Guillaume, and Burt Lancaster. Add to this boxer Rocky Graziano and musician Miles Davis. Not to mention, former presidents Richard Nixon, Gerald Ford, and Dwight Eisenhower. This list could go on and on, and in fact will go on and on, until we improve in the field of stroke prevention.

However, stroke is not just a disease of the rich and famous; it happens all too commonly. In the United States, approximately 700,000 people suffer new strokes every year. Stroke is the third most common cause of death in the United States and in most other developed countries. Just as significantly, if not more so, stroke is the leading cause of disability. Stroke patients' ability to recover varies from complete recovery to death and everything else that is possible in between those two extremes. This is why stroke is such an important health topic and something feared by so many people of all ages.

Over the past ten to fifteen years, doctors and scientists have put increasing resources at learning more about stroke. One popular notion is to rename stroke as "brain attack." This term better conveys exactly what a stroke is: a serious medical emergency involving the brain. Also over the past ten to fifteen years, doctors have found and tested new and innovative treatments for stroke. Twenty years ago, there were no effective treatments for stroke and few large studies to test new treatments. Science has made some progress since then, but there is much more that needs to be accomplished in regard to the prevention and treatment of stroke.

Over the course of the next several chapters, we will learn more about stroke. In the next chapter, we will discuss just who is at risk for strokes and who has them. Before we tackle that problem, however, we need to better understand the circulation of blood flow in the body because, without this knowledge, one cannot understand the pathophysiology of stroke.

The heart is a muscular organ that pumps blood to the entire body. Figure 1.1 summarizes the relevant anatomy that is important for the reader to understand. Blood returning from the tissues by way of the veins enters the right

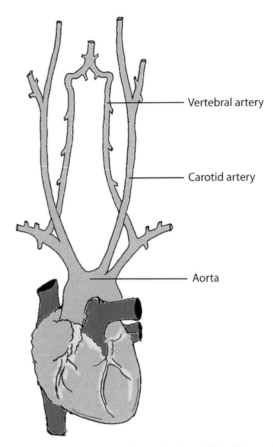

Vertebral artery

Carotid artery

Aorta

Figure 1.1. Illustration of the blood flow from the heart. Blood leaves the left ventricle of the heart and enters the aorta. From the aorta and its branches, the four arteries that supply blood to the brain exit. There are two paired arteries: the right and left carotid arteries and the right and left vertebral arteries. These four blood vessels form a circle at the base of the brain (see Figure 1.2).

side of the heart and is then pumped to the lungs so that oxygen can be replenished. The oxygen-rich blood returns to the left side of the heart and is then released from the left ventricle. It then flows into the major blood vessel of the body: the aorta. All of the major branch arteries that supply blood to the entire body come off the aorta. For example, the mesenteric artery supplies the intestines, the femoral arteries supply the legs, the hepatic artery supplies the liver, the renal artery supplies the kidneys, and so forth. Of importance to understanding stroke is the cerebrovascular circulation, the four arteries that supply blood flow to the brain.

The two largest arteries that branch off the aorta are called the carotid arteries. These large arteries in the front of the neck supply blood to the front (or anterior) part of the brain. The carotid arteries and their branches are called the "anterior circulation." The two smaller arteries in the back of the neck are the vertebral arteries. These two blood vessels supply the back, or "posterior circulation," of the brain. All of these arteries join at the base of the brain in a circular structure called the Circle of Willis (see Figure 1.1), which was named after the seventeenth-century English anatomist Thomas Willis, who first described this web of blood vessels.

This circular structure is an important illustration of nature's wisdom. If any one of the major four arteries in the neck becomes blocked, the other three can take over to supply blood via the Circle of Willis. This concept, called "collateral circulation," in which arteries support each other if the first becomes blocked, is an important one and happens in most of the major organs of the body. Figure 1.2 illustrates this concept of collateral circulation. Subsequent chapters will discuss this concept in greater detail.

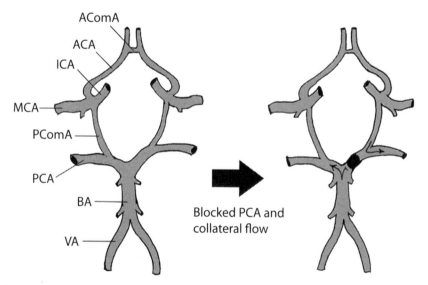

Figure 1.2. The left panel illustrates the Circle of Willis. ICA, internal carotid artery; VA, vertebral artery. These are the four vessels that are seen in Figure 1.2. They form a circle at the base of the brain, and all of the arteries supplying blood to the brain come from this circle. AComA, anterior communicating artery; ACA, anterior cerebral artery; MCA, middle cerebral artery; PComA, posterior communicating artery; BA, basilar artery. The communicating arteries are what form the circle. The right panel shows how collateral circulation works. Blood flows around the circle to bypass the blockage so that flow to that portion of the brain is preserved.

The venous side of the circulation is also important. Venous refers to the veins, whereas arterial refers to the arteries. The difference between veins and arteries lies in what they pump. Arteries contain oxygen-rich blood that flows away from the heart, whereas veins return oxygen-poor blood from the tissues back to the heart. Blood enters the brain, passes from the larger arteries into progressively smaller blood vessels, and finally into capillaries. It is here, at the capillary level, in the brain as in the rest of the body, where the real action occurs. Oxygen, glucose, and other nutrients cross from the capillary and enter the brain cells. Carbon dioxide and other waste products leave the brain cells and enter the capillaries to be returned to the right side of the heart by way of the venous system.

The veins of the brain start small and then coalesce into progressively larger veins. These large veins join together in several places in the brain to form large venous sinuses, or cerebral venous sinuses. These sinuses ultimately direct the blood to the jugular veins, which in turn lead the blood to the right side of the heart. The right side of the heart pumps blood to the lungs, where oxygen and carbon dioxide are exchanged again (this time, the carbon dioxide going out of the body in exhaled air and oxygen entering the blood from inspired air). The blood from the lungs then flows to the left atrium, moves on to the left ventricle, and then out the aorta, where the cycle starts anew.

Tedy Bruschi and Sharon Stone had excellent outcomes from their strokes; this is not always the case. For Israeli Prime Minister Ariel Sharon, the outcome was much different. On December 18, 2005, he was rushed to the hospital with weakness. Diagnostic testing showed that he had suffered a small stroke, and he was subsequently treated with blood-thinning medications. Less than a month later, Sharon, who was seventy-seven years old at the time, returned to the hospital, again by ambulance and again complaining of weakness. This time, however, his brain scan showed a cerebral hemorrhage, bleeding in the brain. It required a six-hour emergency surgery to stop the bleeding and stabilize his condition. Even with the surgery, he was left in a coma-like state. He later required a second surgical procedure, and a year and a half after that, he remains in a coma with dim chances of any meaningful recovery.

We can see that stroke is an important disease of the twenty-first century, of young and old, men and women, celebrities and average citizens. In the next chapters, we will examine why some people are at higher risk of stroke than others and the symptoms of stroke. Succeeding chapters will discuss how doctors diagnose and treat stroke patients and various methods to try to prevent strokes from occurring. Last, we will examine the long-term outcomes of stroke victims to get a better perspective on how the lives of Tedy Bruschi, Sharon Stone, and Ariel Sharon will be affected. The closing chapter will discuss new approaches that are currently being researched to improve stroke care.

2

Pathophysiology and Risk Factors for Stroke

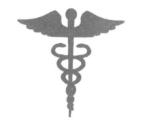

We know that 700,000 persons each year have a stroke in the United States. An important question for all people, their families, and their doctors is who will have a stroke and who will not. Although medical science is not so advanced as to be able to answer that question at the level of individual patients, doctors have learned a lot about which groups of patients are at risk for stroke.

As we alluded to in Chapter 1, there are different risk factors for patients with ischemic (blood clot that impedes flow) vs. hemorrhagic (blood that has escaped from a vessel) stroke, so we will discuss them separately. To properly explore the notion of risk factors, this concept of stroke subtypes needs to be fleshed out a bit more at this point. Understanding how doctors divide strokes into various categories is crucial to understanding the subsequent chapters in this book. The risk factors are different depending on the type of stroke. Although there is overlap, some of the symptoms vary. Diagnostic testing, especially the most important brain imaging test, the CAT scan, shows very different results in the major two groups.

Doctors classify different types of stroke based on their "pathophysiology." The pathophysiology of any disease is how the normal physiology is altered by a disease, or pathologic, process. Dividing strokes into ischemic and

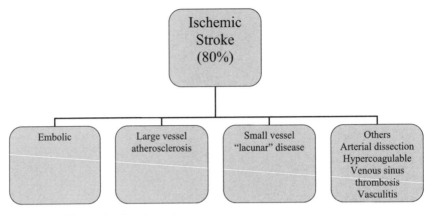

Figure 2.1. Types of ischemic stroke.

hemorrhagic is based on their different pathophysiology. Further subdividing them into more precise stroke subtypes is based on their different pathophysiology. It makes sense then that different types of strokes have different risk factors.

Ischemic stroke, strokes caused by clots that block blood flow, is by far the most common and accounts for approximately 80 percent of all strokes. There are a number of subtypes of ischemic stroke (see Figure 2.1). Hemorrhagic strokes account for the remaining 20 percent of strokes, and, again, several subtypes exist (see Figure 2.2).

At first glance, this may seem complicated, but it's not. Let's first focus on ischemic strokes.

The underlying process in an ischemic stroke is the blockage of blood flow to a portion of the brain that is normally supplied by the affected artery. There

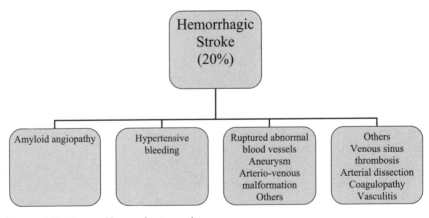

Figure 2.2. Types of hemorrhagic stroke.

are a number of ways that this can happen. An "embolism" is a blood clot that forms in one part of the body and then travels (or embolizes) to another area in the body, and an embolic stroke is one in which a blood clot travels from one place in the body to another. Of course, all of this happens within blood vessels. The end result is death of brain cells as a result of lack of oxygen and glucose. The symptoms may differ depending on which part of the brain is involved.

There are many causes of brain ischemia; let's examine the most important examples.

EMBOLIC STROKE RESULTING FROM HEART DISEASE

The most common cause of embolism occurs in a heart (cardiac) condition called "atrial fibrillation." Normally, each electrical impulse causes the atria (upper chambers of the heart) to beat in a strong, coordinated, and efficient manner. The blood flows smoothly. In atrial fibrillation, there are no coordinated electrical impulses, and therefore there is no coordinated mechanical pumping of blood in the atria. When this occurs over long periods of time (usually weeks to months or even longer), clots form in these upper chambers of the heart. Sometimes, these clots will dislodge and travel from the heart into the aorta and up the carotid or vertebral artery. The clot can then lodge in one of these arteries or in one of their branches, which will cause a stroke.

Other cardiac problems besides atrial fibrillation can lead to clots that can embolize to the brain. Clots can also form in the ventricles (the lower chambers of the heart) after a heart attack. Patients with dilated ventricles from any cause, such as "cardiomyopathy," left ventricular aneurysm, or congestive heart failure, are also at risk for developing clot and therefore are at higher than average risk for stroke. The common denominator of all three of these conditions is that the heart is dilated or swollen and there is sluggish blood flow. Both of these factors promote the blood to clot.

There are other places where clots can form that can also embolize to the brain, the aorta and carotid artery being the most common. So, atherosclerosis in these two locations can result in stroke. As the population ages and baby-boomers reach the ages when atherosclerosis becomes more prevalent, doctors are increasingly recognizing atherosclerotic plaque in the aorta as a risk factor for stroke.

One unusual but not rare cause of stroke is known as "paradoxical embolism." In this condition, the clot forms in the venous side of the circulation, usually in the veins of the legs. This is called a deep venous thrombosis (DVT). This clot can migrate, or embolize, to the heart. Normally, it crosses

Table 2.1.
Risk Factors for Embolic Stroke

Atrial fibrillation
Atherosclerosis of the aorta and carotid arteries
Heart attack
Cardiomyopathy
Left ventricular aneurysm
PFO
Endocarditis

the right atrium and right ventricle and enters the lung, a condition called pulmonary embolism. However, 20 percent of individuals have a connection between the right and left atria. This is called a "patent foramen ovale" (PFO) and is a remnant of a normal structure in the growing fetus that simply never disappeared in some people. If a clot from a DVT travels to the heart and crosses a PFO, it can then travel to one of the carotid or vertebral arteries and cause a stroke. This is exactly what happened to Tedy Bruschi. Although the source of his clot was never found for certain, it almost certainly crossed a PFO that doctors found on his diagnostic testing, causing a paradoxical embolism.

Another cardiac condition that is associated with embolic stroke is called endocarditis. This is an infection in the lining of the heart (or endocardium). The infection causes clumps of bacteria and inflammatory debris to form on the heart valves. These clumps of material, called vegetations, can embolize to the brain and cause a stroke. This is a relatively unusual cause but an important one to diagnose because the treatments will be different. A full discussion of endocarditis is beyond the scope of this book, but, simply stated, if bacteria gain access to the bloodstream, they can lodge and start growing on the valves in the heart. This usually happens only with an already abnormal valve. Once the heart valve infection starts, vegetations made up of blood platelets and bacteria can grow and then embolize to the brain, causing a stroke. Table 2.1 summarizes the important risk factors for embolic strokes.

ATHEROSCLEROSIS

The next major subcategory of ischemic stroke is large-vessel atherosclerosis, which is the pathological process in the body whereby plaques containing cholesterol and other blood components form in arteries. This leads to partial or complete blockages in the arteries that decrease the flow of blood distally.

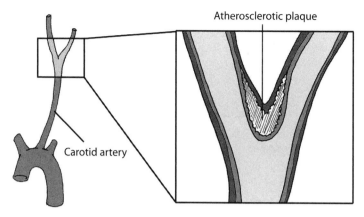

Figure 2.3. The typical location of an atherosclerotic plaque. As the plaque enlarges, it begins to block blood flow. When it reaches 50–60 percent obstruction, flow is usually decreased. Sometimes, because of the collateral circulation afforded by the Circle of Willis (see Figure 1.2), there is no problem; other times, a blocked carotid leads to brain ischemia.

The most important location for atherosclerosis as it leads to stroke is the carotid artery.

The carotid arteries (there is one on each side) arise from the aorta. The carotid artery splits, or bifurcates, in the neck into the external and internal carotid arteries. The internal carotid artery is the one that supplies the brain. Atherosclerosis often forms at branch points in arteries (bifurcations). Thus, a common place for an atherosclerotic plaque to form is this bifurcation, where the common carotid artery splits into the internal and external. Figure 2.3 shows a schematic of what this looks like. You can see that, as the plaque gets larger and larger, it blocks a progressively larger percentage of the "lumen" of the blood vessel. The more the blockage in the internal carotid artery (carotid artery stenosis), the less the blood flows; therefore, higher degrees of internal carotid artery stenosis is a risk factor for ischemic stroke.

Risk factors for atherosclerosis are much the same for heart and other cardiovascular disorders: cigarette smoking, high blood pressure (or "hypertension"), diabetes sedentary lifestyle, and elevated blood lipids (such as cholesterol and "triglycerides). However, genetic factors play a role as well. Genes are bits of DNA that code for proteins to be synthesized. Some genetic factors, for example, race or sex, are obvious from the outside; others, such as the chemical makeup of a particular protein in the body, are much less obvious.

GENETIC FACTORS

Although we currently cannot modify genetic risk factors, that possibility exists in the future as we learn more about gene modification. Some genetic factors are easy to find. Race is the most obvious one. The mortality rate of stroke is much higher in blacks than in whites. Using data from 2001, the mortality rate of stroke in black men was about 85 percent, whereas the rate for white males was 55 percent. Some of this could be attributable to access to healthcare but certainly not the whole discrepancy.

Other genetic factors are less obvious. Gene mutations for a variety of proteins increase the risk of both ischemic and hemorrhagic stroke.

ELEVATED LIPIDS

There are two important blood lipids: cholesterol and triglycerides. Cholesterol is a critical component of cell walls, and, without some of it, we would die. Similarly, triglycerides are essential to forming cell walls. Like many things in life, cholesterol and triglycerides are essential to have, but, if the levels are excessive, they can lead to problems. Elevated cholesterol and triglycerides lead to accelerated atherosclerosis, because these two substances become part of the atherosclerotic plaque that blocks arteries. Simply put, elevated blood lipids are an important risk factor for large-vessel atherosclerosis that causes stroke.

SMALL-VESSEL DISEASE

Small-vessel disease is also called "lacunar" stroke. The small vessels in the brain refer to the small-sized arteries that penetrate into the base of the brain. They originate from larger arteries that make up the Circle of Willis and supply blood flow to small areas of the brain toward the bottom of the brain. Strokes involving these small penetrating vessels lead to strokes involving small but critical areas of the brain. If a patient with a lacunar stroke dies (often from some other cause) and has an autopsy, the area of stroke looks to the pathologist like a tiny lake embedded in the normal tissue. Lacunar stroke gets its name because the Latin word for lake is "lacune."

Risk factors for small-vessel disease, also called "lipohyalinosis" because of the appearance of these blood vessels under a microscope, are similar to those for large-vessel disease. Table 2.2 shows the risk factors for both large-vessel and small-vessel disease. Advancing age is an independent risk factor for stroke, as we shall discuss later in this chapter in more detail.

Table 2.2.
Risk Factors for Large-Vessel and Small-Vessel Disease

Diabetes
Hypertension
Cigarette smoking
Elevated cholesterol and triglycerides
Carotid artery stenosis
Sedentary lifestyle
Genetic factors
Age

These first three categories, embolic, large-vessel, and small-vessel disease, account for the large majority of ischemic strokes. However, there are other pathological conditions that can also result in ischemic stroke. One of them is arterial dissection. Arteries have three layers: the outer layer (adventitia), a middle muscular layer (muscularis), and a delicate inside layer called the intima. Sometimes, blood will enter tiny tears in the intima and begin to split (or dissect) the layers of the artery, peeling the intima from the muscular layer or the muscular layer from the adventitia. This is an arterial dissection. The blood within the layers of the artery can cause a narrowing of the lumen of the artery. The narrowing leads to stroke if the blockage sufficiently reduces flow, usually by more than 80–90 percent. Dissections can occur in either the carotid or the vertebral artery and rarely in more than one artery at the same time. Hypertension is a risk factor for arterial dissection, as are various diseases of connective tissue, which are the tissues that make up the various layers of the arteries. Table 2.3 lists the risk factors for arterial dissections.

BLOOD COAGULATION

Hypercoagulable states are another unusual cause of stroke. There is a constant interplay in the body between factors that cause the blood to clot, or coagulate, and factors that cause the blood to remain liquid. Having these two competing systems may seem odd at first, but consider the following situation. You accidentally cut your finger while opening a tin can. If there were no mechanism in the body to stop this bleeding, you could bleed to death from a simple laceration. In fact, when the body senses bleeding, it begins to limit the blood loss. The blood vessels go into spasm. Proteins in the blood called clotting factors are activated, which form a clot inside the blood vessels. Last, solid elements in the blood called platelets also get into the act to make a solid plug in the torn blood vessel. The clotting factors and platelets are very

Table 2.3.
Risk Factors for Hemorrhagic Stroke

Increasing age
High blood pressure
Anticoagulant and anti-platelet medications
Cerebral aneurysms
  High blood pressure
  Binge alcohol drinking
  Cigarette smoking
  Genetic factors
  Family history of ruptured aneurysms
AVM
Any condition that leads to diminished ability of blood clotting
  Intrinsic: medical conditions such as hemophilia or liver disease
  Iatrogenic: anticoagulant medications
Drug abuse (cocaine, amphetamines, diet pills, and others)
Other miscellaneous blood vessel abnormalities

important, as we will see in the chapter on prevention and treatment of stroke.

This clotting mechanism is all well and good, but if it were not for a similar balancing mechanism to tell the body when to stop clotting, all the flow in the body could stop from one huge clot. So there are mechanisms in the body to break up, or "lyse," clot. This is a competing system called the thrombolytic (clot breaking) system that is a cascade of enzymes and proteins whose job it is to break up clot that is not benefiting the body at any given time.

These two systems, the coagulation and thrombolytic systems, are in constant interplay in the body to get things just right. As Goldilocks might say, "not too much clotting, not too much thrombolysis." However, there are times when this competition is thrown out of balance. When the procoagulant side of the equation is stronger, then the body tends to form clot when it is not needed; this is called a "hypercoagulable" state. When the anticoagulant side overpowers, the body tends to bleed too easily; this is called a coagulopathy.

Patients who are hypercoagulable have a tendency to have ischemic strokes, but, because the tendency is all over the body, they can also have clotting problems in any area of the body. There is a long list of conditions that lead to this state. Most are problems with the various proteins that help with blood coagulation: deficiencies with protein S, protein C, and antithrombin III, a mutant type of prothrombin gene, and of a blood coagulation factor called Factor V Leiden (named after the city in Holland where it was first described). These are just a few; there are others that have been identified. In addition, some of these factors have only recently been identified. Because some patients who seem to form frequent blood clots go without a clear cause, it is likely that others will be discovered in the future.

One important and common factor that is known is the use of estrogen-containing birth control pills. The first generation of oral contraceptives had high levels of estrogens, and women who took them were found to have higher risk of stroke and heart attack. Over time, the estrogen contents of the pills have gotten lower and lower, but there is still some risk associated with birth control pills, especially in women who also smoke cigarettes and have migraine headaches. This latter factor, migraines, may be a risk for stroke in its own right.

A related problem to generalized hypercoagulability is the problem of cerebral venous sinus thrombosis (CVST). We have already talked about a DVT or clot in a leg vein. CVST is just like a DVT of the brain. In fact, the risk factors for both DVT and CVST are similar. We have talked about how stroke is caused by a decreased supply of nutrients to the brain because of an arterial problem, and CVST is one exception to this definition. Stroke specialists include CVST as a cause of stroke, but it breaks a lot of the usual rules. For one, it is a problem with the venous side of the brain circulation, not of the arterial side. Second, the symptoms tend to be a little different because the pattern of brain dysfunction does not follow the usual arterial territory patterns. Last, as you may have noticed from the charts at the beginning of the chapter, CVST can lead to both ischemic and hemorrhagic strokes.

Vasculitis is the inflammation of a blood vessel, usually of an artery or arteries. This inflammation usually happens for unclear reasons, but evidence suggests that immunological factors play an important role. In some cases, the inflammation causes thrombosis within an artery; this thrombosis can decrease distal blood flow and cause stroke. Most strokes from vasculitis are ischemic, but, as in CVST, some strokes from vasculitis are hemorrhagic.

All of these stroke subtypes discussed above account for the vast majority of ischemic strokes.

The unifying pathophysiology of hemorrhagic strokes is that blood escapes from the inside of blood vessels. Understanding hemorrhagic strokes requires knowing another basic fact of neuroanatomy. The brain is enclosed in a rigid bony box, the skull. Inside this bony structure sits the brain, blood inside of blood vessels, and cerebrospinal fluid (CSF). If pressure increases inside the skull, something has to give. The brain itself is not very compressible, neither is the blood, although to an extent, both venous and arterial blood can be pushed out of the skull. Higher pressure can compress the veins and arteries so that blood, still inside the blood vessels, is displaced to blood vessels outside the skull. Last, the CSF (also not compressible) can be displaced into the CSF space along the spine.

In hemorrhagic stroke, blood enters the intracranial space. Without these compensatory mechanisms, this increase in volume (of blood) would be expected to increase the pressure in this closed space (the skull, or intracranial space). If the volume of blood that has escaped is small, the compensatory mechanisms work to blunt the rise in intracranial pressure (ICP) that would otherwise occur. However, each of the compensatory mechanisms to blunt a rise in ICP, displacement of venous blood, arterial blood, and CSF, is limited. As increasing amounts of blood enter the intracranial space, at some point in time, the compensatory mechanisms are overwhelmed, and the ICP rises rapidly.

This rise in ICP leads to shifts of brain structures, called herniation, then to (initially) reversible neurological dysfunction and later, irreversible brain dysfunction, and finally brain death. In addition to the blood creating a mass effect from elevated pressure and volume, blood is irritating to the brain, so swelling and inflammation also occur, which creates even more volume and pressure. Last, sometimes blood that enters the CSF can irritate the blood vessels that run along the surface of the brain. This irritation can lead to spasm, and the spasm can lead to ischemia. Therefore, in some kinds of hemorrhagic stroke, an element of ischemia also contributes to the brain dysfunction.

Now let's shift our attention to the pathophysiology of the more common types of hemorrhagic stroke.

HEMORRHAGIC STROKE

Major Types

Amyloid angiopathy is a big name, but it is easier if it is broken down into parts. Angiopathy comes from "angio" (blood vessel) and "pathy" or disease. Amyloid is a chemical substance. So the fancy word just means a disease of blood vessels that is caused by this chemical deposition. The infiltration of amyloid occurs most commonly in the blood vessels in the brains of much older individuals, which is why this condition is being seen more often as Americans live longer and longer. At some point, especially if the blood pressure is a bit high, blood will leak out from a spot in a brain artery that has been weakened by the amyloid and spill over into the brain substance. So, age is a risk factor. Although there is no specific age cutoff, the likelihood of developing this problem increases dramatically in individuals over seventy years of age.

Hypertensive bleeds into the brain is another important category of hemorrhagic stroke. Elevated blood pressure, especially at high levels for long periods of time, can weaken small blood vessels and lead to rupture with bleeding into the brain. High blood pressure can also cause bleeding in an area of abnormal blood vessels (such as an aneurysm). Fortunately, hypertensive bleeding is becoming much less common over time. As physicians and public health campaigns have improved high blood pressure care in America, the incidence of this form of bleeding has decreased considerably over the past few decades.

Although hypertensive bleeds are decreasing, another form of hemorrhagic stroke is on the increase. This is bleeding related to anticoagulation therapy. Ironically, some of these anticoagulant drugs are prescribed to prevent ischemic stroke. The major offender here is Coumadin, also referred to as the generic form warfarin. This medication renders the blood thinner, making the blood less likely to clot. There is a narrow range of safety with this drug: too little and the patient is not protected, but just a little too much and the patient is at risk of bleeding. Not only is the dosage tricky, but other medications and even various foods can throw off the correct dose. As expected, the most important side-effect is bleeding, including bleeding in the brain. Because more patients are being treated with blood thinners, hemorrhagic strokes are on the rise. Until safer alternatives are found, this increase will likely continue into the next decade or longer. In addition, other medications that thin the blood, from simple aspirin and other more potent anti-platelet medications, also contribute to the burden of hemorrhagic stroke. Less commonly, some patients will have poor clotting as a result of other medical conditions, such as liver disease or nutritional problems. These conditions, too, can result in bleeding in the brain.

Aneurysm and Arteriovenous Malformation

Another group of conditions that lead to hemorrhagic stroke are various abnormal blood vessels that may rupture. The most common is the cerebral aneurysm. An aneurysm is a weak spot in an artery, sort of like a weak spot in a tire that balloons out. If you pump more air into that tire, eventually the weak spot will break and the air rapidly leaves the tire. The same thing happens in aneurysms. Aneurysms can occur in any artery in the body. Typical locations include the aorta and the cerebral blood vessels. In the latter case, the weak points are typically at the places where brain arteries branch at and near the Circle of Willis.

Minor Types

Other conditions also cause bleeding in the brain, and, although not very common, all are important because treatments exist for them. In venous sinus thrombosis, clot forms in the veins that drain the brain. Paradoxically, sometimes these clotted veins (or the venous sinuses that they drain into) will rupture and cause bleeding. This condition is caused by a long list of things that also predispose to venous clotting in the veins of the legs, which is a much more common condition.

Other times, various medical conditions will cause the blood to be "too thin," meaning that blood does not clot properly, the same as what Coumadin and the blood thinners do. Two examples of this are hemophilia, in which the body does not make sufficient clotting factor X, and liver disease, in which the liver does not make a variety of clotting factors. In both of these conditions, very minor trauma can precipitate life-threatening bleeding.

Yet another condition is called an arterial dissection. We discussed this condition earlier in the chapter to show that it could lead to decreased blood flow (and an ischemic stroke), but it can also rupture and result in a hemorrhagic stroke. In fact, this was the etiology of actress Sharon Stone's hemorrhage. Another unusual condition called vasculitis, or inflammation of blood vessels, can also occur in brain arteries and result in bleeding. Although all of the last several causes are somewhat unusual, all have effective treatments so doctors must consider them in patients who present with hemorrhagic strokes.

There is even a geographical factor: the so-called "stroke belt." This is a multi-state area in the southeastern United States where the risk for and mortality rate from stroke are higher than in the remainder of the country. This phenomenon was first noticed several decades ago, and researchers are still trying to sort out the cause. Are there environmental factors? Genetic factors? Does it relate to the quality of medical care or access to medical care? Or perhaps cultural factors such as dietary or smoking habits, or economic factors such as poverty? The reality is that we simply do not know for certain, but most likely this phenomenon has to do with a complex combination of many (if not all) of these factors.

There is one other general way of thinking about risk factors for just about any disease. Are the risks modifiable or not? Let's examine two of the most obvious examples: age and cigarette smoking. One cannot change one's age; a sixty-year-old man cannot make himself forty. However, a cigarette smoker can and should stop smoking.

Table 2.4 lists the American Heart Association's (AHA) list of modifiable and nonmodifiable risk factors for stroke.

There are also factors whose contributions are not entirely clear as of yet. Some examples include homocysteine and folate levels. The first, an amino acid, and the second, a vitamin, may both play a role in heart disease and stroke. The role of inflammation in the body is another example of this. Some physicians will measure the "C-reactive protein" level in their patients' blood

Table 2.4.
Risk Factors for Stroke (modifiable and nonmodifiable)

Nonmodifiable
   Age
   Sex
   Genetic factors
   Previous TIA and heart and other cardiovascular disease
Modifiable
   High blood pressure
   Diabetes
   Cigarette smoking
   Carotid artery disease
   Arterial fibrillation
   Other forms of heart disease (PFO, cardiomyopathy, and valvular heart disease)
   Dietary factors and obesity
   Sedentary lifestyle
   Hypercoagulable states
   Sickle cell disease
   Elevated cholesterol
   Heavy alcohol use (for subarachnoid hemorrhage)
   Drug abuse (for some kinds of stroke)

---

to try to predict risk for cardiovascular problems. There are almost certainly other factors that we don't yet know about or about which our level of understanding is not yet well developed. Hopefully, learning more about risk factors will increase doctors' ability to prevent stroke.

So although the bad news is that some risk factors (age, sex, genetic background, and past medical events) cannot be changed, the large majority, and very important ones, can be. Changing lifestyle (diet, smoking, and exercise), treating medical conditions (lowering blood pressure, treating serious carotid artery disease), as well as many others can lower one's risk of stroke.

3

Symptoms: Am I Having a Stroke?

W e go about day-to-day activities and take for granted the normal function of our bodies. We do not think about our hearts beating, our lungs breathing, or our brains functioning.

Therefore, when we suddenly lose one of those functions, or somehow become focused on them, the resulting situation can be quite frightening.

One of the hallmarks of a stroke, implied in the very word, is the sudden onset of symptoms. One second a person is normal, and the next is marked by some part of the body simply not responding to the usual commands being sent out from the brain. Recall that the three elements of a stroke have to do with (1) abrupt onset, (2) symptoms attributable to loss of blood flow in a single arterial territory, and (3) the duration of symptoms last at least twenty-four hours. Let's focus on each of these elements separately.

ABRUPT ONSET

The sudden onset of symptoms helps to distinguish stroke from other neurological problems that can be confused with stroke. The weakness from a brain tumor could be the same as the weakness caused by a stroke, but the former usually begins slowly and progresses over time whereas the weakness from a stroke begins suddenly. The visual losses from a cataract, or an infection in the eye, also manifest themselves gradually, whereas the decreased vision from a stroke (or a TIA) begins abruptly.

Therefore, this type of onset is very helpful to doctors in distinguishing the cause of one kind of neurological dysfunction from another. It is important to recognize, however, that some patients with stroke, especially the ischemic kind, may go to sleep normal and wake up with their neurological deficit. In this setting, although the precise time of onset cannot be firmly established, we presume that the neurological deficit began at some specific point in time during the night.

NEUROLOGICAL DYSFUNCTION IN A SINGLE ARTERIAL TERRITORY

This component of the definition of stroke is also important in helping to define the condition. This is especially true in an ischemic stroke. If one artery has lost blood flow, the brain tissue that is supplied by that artery either ceases to function or functions poorly. The patient will have particular symptoms. We will explore this concept further later in this chapter, but a patient with a left middle cerebral artery clot will have different symptoms than a patient with a right anterior cerebral artery clot. That is to say, the particular symptoms that an individual patient has are attributable to which part of the brain is not working correctly.

In a hemorrhage, some of the symptoms can be a result of pressure on more remote areas of the brain the nonspecific irritation caused by blood in the CSF. However, when there is a hematoma that has leaked into the brain tissue itself, the symptoms will be more or less focal based on which part of the brain is involved.

DURATION OF SYMPTOMS LASTS GREATER THAN TWENTY-FOUR HOURS

The final factor relates to how long the symptoms last. The classic distinction between a TIA and a stroke has to do with this factor of duration. However, this distinction has become less important over the past decade for several reasons.

First, because there are treatments for acute ischemic stroke that have to be given within a very short period of time, in fact within three hours of onset, having a twenty-four-hour time distinction simply doesn't make sense any more. Second, as doctors do magnetic resonance imaging (MRI) scans on more patients whose symptoms do not last twenty-four hours, they are finding that some of the patients whose symptoms have gone away have actually had a stroke (more about this in the next chapter). For both of these reasons, for patients who see their doctors in the first hours after symptom onset, the time duration is a less important part of the definition than the first two components.

SPECIFIC SYMPTOMS

The specific symptoms in a given patient relate to several factors. First and foremost is the part of the brain involved by this stroke. Chapter 1 introduced the Circle of Willis, the arterial rotary at the base of the brain off which various branches extend. To properly understand stroke symptoms, one must first understand three important facts of neuroanatomy. The first is the Circle of Willis and its major branches. The second crucial concept has to do with some basic wiring of the brain. The third is the fact that different parts of the brain are the centers for different functions.

Recall from Chapter 1 that there are four major arteries: two carotid arteries and two vertebral arteries that travel upward in the neck to bring the brain its blood supply that contains glucose and oxygen. These four arteries hook into a circle, or rotary, at the base of the brain called the Circle of Willis. The importance of this circular design is that, if one of the major arteries in the neck is blocked, blood from the other three arteries may be able to supply enough collateral blood flow to the brain to avoid a stroke.

This circle is divided into the front part of the circulation (the anterior circulation) and the back part (the posterior circulation). In the anterior circulation, the carotid artery divides into three major arteries: the ophthalmic, the anterior cerebral, and the middle cerebral arteries. In the posterior circulation, the vertebral arteries join to form the large basilar artery, which gives rise to arteries to the cerebellum, the brainstem, and the posterior cerebral artery.

It is not important to memorize this right now, but it is critical to know that a stroke involving one part of the brain will lead to symptoms that are completely different from those of a stroke involving another part. The second critical fact to know has to do with how the brain and its connections are wired to the spinal cord. There are areas in the nervous system in which large cables of neurons switch sides from right to left or vice versa.

Overall, brain anatomy goes something like this (see Figure 3.1). The cerebrum is the most developed (and highest) portion of the brain. It is large in humans and progressively smaller in more primitive animals. Nerve fibers from the cerebrum descend and are funneled into the internal capsule, an area dense in fibers, some of which stop at a relay station called the thalamus. These nerve fibers then descend lower to the brainstem, which is divided into three portions. From upper to lower are the midbrain, the pons, and the

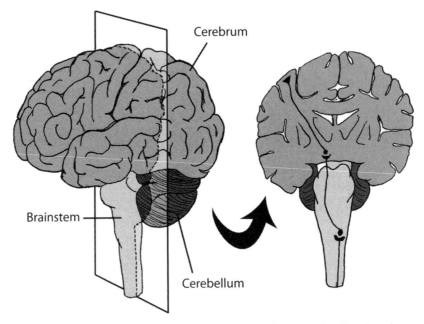

Figure 3.1. Basic brain anatomy. The cerebrum is the most developed in human beings, and different parts are for different functions. The cerebellum is the part of the brain that is important for balance and coordination. All of the tracts of nerves that go from these first two structures to the body (by way of the spinal cord) travel through the brainstem. The clusters of nerve cells that form the nucleus for the cranial nerves are also located in the brainstem.

medulla. The cerebellum (not to be confused with the cerebrum) lies over the top of the brainstem. At the point at which the head becomes the neck, the medulla becomes the spinal cord, which descends in the bony spine and sends out nerves that control the muscles and receive sensation from the body.

Thus, a stroke involving the right side of the brain will result in a deficit of the left side of the body, and a stroke involving the left side of the brain will affect the right side of the body. So the symptoms in any individual patient are mostly affected by which artery is involved and which side of the brain is involved. The majority of these cables of nerve fibers cross in the brainstem, a portion of the brain that connects the upper brain (cerebrum) to the spinal cord. The brainstem contains many cells of the nerves called the cranial nerves. These nerves, for the most part, supply motor and sensory function to various structures in the head and upper neck. A stroke that occurs in the brainstem may affect the face and neck on the same side as the stroke but the arms and legs on the opposite side.

A stroke of the cerebellum usually affects the same side of the body. Although this can get confusing, it is not important to know the details at this point. What is important is to know that the specific parts of the body that are involved give important clues about what portion of the brain is affected. With that background, we can now talk about stroke symptoms.

The third important fact is that different lobes of the brain are the centers for different functions. For example, the frontal lobes are relatively silent in terms of acute stroke symptoms, at least with regard to weakness or sensory findings. The right parietal lobe tends to be important with spatial relationships, whereas its counterpart on the left is the speech center. The back part, or occipital lobes, is important for vision and interpreting what we see. The cerebellum is the center of balance; as you might imagine, this part of the brain is very well developed in cats and birds.

As mentioned above, the brainstem is an area of brain that connects the cerebrum to the spinal cord.

The brainstem is densely packed with nerve bundles that descend from brain to spinal cord (for example, telling the saxophonist's fingers to move to play different notes) and others that ascend from cord to brain (for example, those from the legs that tell the brain the exact position at any given moment of the right foot). The brainstem also contains important clusters of nerve cells that control eye movement, mouth and face sensation, and muscle activity. As the marching band member strolls down the field, the muscles that control the eyes allow him to read the notes on the sheet of music and other nerves fire to make his mouth achieve just the right tension to play a given note.

Ultimately, all these different parts of the body are represented in different locations of the brain that is best illustrated by the "homunculus." This is the distorted picture of different body parts as they are represented along the surface of the brain. Sometimes, larger areas of brain control smaller parts of the body, such as the tongue, mouth, and thumb, which are anatomically small but functionally important. Figure 3.2 shows the homunculus. There is a homunculus for motor activity and another for sensory activity. They lie side by side in the cerebrum, the upper part of the brain.

In an ischemic stroke, a clot blocks flow of blood distal to where the clot sits. The portion of the brain that normally received nutrients from the artery stops functioning. Therefore, whatever functions that part of the brain controls instantly stop. So if a person were to have a clot lodge in the right middle cerebral artery, they would have the onset of left-sided weakness and numbness. Because this part of the brain is also responsible for spatial relations, sometimes these patients will not recognize someone standing to their left. In addition, they may awake lying in the bed diagonally. A clot blocking flow to

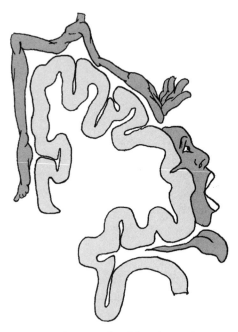

Figure 3.2. Illustration of the homunculus. This shows the representation of various body parts on the cerebral cortex. Note that the face, lips, and tongue get a lot of territory in the brain, although they are relatively small in size. The same is true of the hand and even the thumb. These parts of the body need a lot of brain tissue to help support their very detailed functions.

the left middle cerebral artery would lead to right-sided weakness and problems with speech, because the left brain is largely responsible for language. This loss of ability to speak is called aphasia.

A stroke of the cerebellum will lead to imbalance and vertigo, the illusory sense of motion in the environment. If large enough, the patient's balance can be so poor that they cannot walk at all. Because the cerebellum lies in a very small and constrained portion of the brain, the posterior fossa, headache is common with this kind of stroke. A stroke involving the anterior cerebral artery would preferentially affect the leg more than the face or the arm because that vessel supplies blood to the middle portion of the brain, where the leg is mostly represented on the homunculus. Thus, a left anterior cerebral artery stroke might involve the right leg more than other body parts on the right.

These are some examples of strokes involving large cerebral blood vessels, but there are also very small "penetrating" arteries that come off the Circle of Willis and the basilar artery. These small penetrating arteries that arise from the circle provide blood supply to some of the deep portions of the brain, such as the "internal capsule." In these areas, the nerve fibers are densely packed so that such strokes can lead to paralysis of face, arm, and leg equally, but they do not affect higher brain functions such as speech or spatial orientation. These strokes affect small amounts of brain tissue but can do a lot of damage because of the amount of neurons that they sometimes affect. When pathologists examine the brains of patients who have died from these smaller strokes, they look like small holes in the brain and are called lacunar strokes.

The penetrating arteries that arise from the basilar artery supply the brainstem, which has a somewhat complicated anatomy. In this critical area, numerous nuclei of the "cranial nerves" sit, and many of the important bundles of nerves pass through. So a brainstem stroke could lead to paralysis of a part of the body and also affect the function of a cranial nerve. Most of the cranial nerves affect function of the face and neck on the same side from which the nerve exits the brain.

Therefore, patients with stroke will present with the abrupt onset of specific neurological deficits that fit with a specific cerebrovascular territory that persists. Table 3.1 illustrates some of the more common stroke syndromes. This table describes the more classic ones, but sometimes patients will not fit a "classic" pattern, either because of variations in their brain vascular anatomy or because not all of a given artery's territory is involved. Sometimes, these same symptoms that occur with a stroke can happen with other entities besides stroke, other conditions called "stroke mimics."

There are a number of things that are important for patients and their families to keep in mind if they are having stroke symptoms. For one, it is important for patients and their families to remember the specific time of onset of the symptoms and to communicate this to the ambulance crew and the medical staff at the ED. This single data point is extremely important to the healthcare providers' decision making with regard to therapy. It is also vitally important to do this immediately. Neither Tedy Bruschi nor Sharon Stone activated 911 immediately. Although both of their cases ended up with favorable results, this is not the norm, and patients or family members should activate 911 rapidly.

One of the pieces of information that the paramedics or emergency medical technicians (EMTs) will get is the time of onset. Another exam that they will do is to quickly assess whether they believe that a stroke is occurring. To do that, they will use one of several pre-hospital stroke scales. The two most common are the Cincinnati stroke scale and the Los Angeles stroke scale (see Table 3.2).

The Cincinnati scale is easy, fast, and very reproducible between different people. If any one of the three measurements is abnormal, there is about a two-thirds chance the patient will have a stroke. This may not sound very accurate, but for a pre-hospital examination that takes all of twenty seconds,

Table 3.1.
Classic Stroke Syndromes

Middle cerebral artery stroke	Unilateral weakness and diminished sensation on the opposite side of the body. The arm and face are more affected than the leg. The eyes often deviate toward the side of the brain involved (and away from the paralyzed side of the body). If the left side is involved, speech is usually abnormal; if the right brain is involved, the patient will not have a good sense of position and will often ignore the left side of his body.
Anterior cerebral artery stroke	Weakness and decreased sensation typically involve the leg only. Because of frontal lobe involvement, some patients will have incontinence, slow thinking, and primitive reflexes such as the suck reflex (patient will make sucking motions if their lips are stimulated). Posterior cerebral artery stroke: hemianopsia (inability to see to the opposite side of the involved brain), often without significant weakness or decreased sensation.
Internal capsule lacunar stroke	Paralysis of the face, arm, and leg, but no sensory loss is seen. In this kind of stroke, the face, arm, and leg are equally affected. Note that, in some internal capsule lacunar stroke, there can be a pure sensory loss (similar to thalamic lacunar stroke; see below).
Thalamic lacunar stroke	A pure sensory stroke occurs with sensory loss in the face, arm, and leg without weakness.
Pontine lacunar stroke	Slurred speech with clumsiness and mild weakness of one arm.
Pontine stroke	If the medial portion of the pons is involved, the lesion produces weakness and an inability to coordinate eye movement (which results in double vision). A lateral pons lesion produces sensory loss and clumsiness of the limbs.
Midbrain stroke	Weber syndrome consists of a dilated pupil, droopy eyelid, and weakness of the muscles that move the eye on the side of the stroke and on the opposite side. Weakness of the body is also found.
Lateral medulla stroke	This results in facial numbness, limb clumsiness, dilated pupil, and droopy eyelid and pain above the eye (on the side of the stroke) with opposite side decreased sensation. Vertigo, nausea, hiccups, hoarseness, difficulty swallowing, and double vision are also found.
Subarachnoid hemorrhage	The classic presentation is the sudden onset of severe headache during activity, associated with a decreased level of consciousness and stiff neck. Because this is usually attributable to a ruptured aneurysm, other neurological symptoms will depend on which artery is involved, but many patients only have the severe headache.
Cerebellar stroke	Headache, vomiting, and inability to walk are typical. Strength and sensation are usually normal. The limbs are typically very clumsy and uncoordinated.

Note: It is important to note that these symptoms listed above are the most common and classic syndromes that occur. There are many exceptions and/or additions seen in actual clinical practice.

Table 3.2.
Pre-hospital Stroke Scales

Cincinnati stroke scale		
Facial droop		
Normal	Both sides of face move equally	
Abnormal	One side of face does not move at all	
Arm drift		
Normal	Both arms move equally or not at all	
Abnormal	One arm drifts compared with the other	
Speech		
Normal	Patient uses correct words with no slurring	
Abnormal	Slurred or inappropriate words or mute	
LA stroke scale		

Screening criteria	Yes	No
Age over 45 years		
No previous history of seizure disorder		
New onset of neurologic symptoms in last 24 hours		
Patient was ambulatory at baseline (before event)		
Blood glucose between 60 and 400		

Exam: look for obvious asymmetry	Normal	Right	Left
Facial smile/grimace		Droop?	Droop?
Grip		Weak grip?	Weak grip?
		No grip?	No grip?
Arm weakness		Drifts down?	Drifts down?
		Falls rapidly?	Falls rapidly?

	Yes	No
Based on exam, patient has only unilateral weakness		

it is actually pretty good, enough so that the ambulance crew will likely alert the ED by radio, a step that can save precious moments at the hospital. The Los Angeles scale is more complicated but also performs well.

If a patient is having a stroke, it is preferable to have them go to the ED by ambulance because patients arriving by ambulance have been shown to get their diagnostic studies done more rapidly and to be treated more quickly if they are eligible to receive some of the treatments that are time sensitive. This is in part because the patients likely arrive to the ED sooner but also because, when the pre-hospital providers notify the ED by radio before their arrival, they are able to swing into action faster than if someone arrives to the ED by private vehicle.

Doctors and nurses in the ED will perform various tests to distinguish between a true stroke and stroke mimics (more about this in Chapter 4).

One exception to the notion of "focal" neurological symptoms is that some patients with an acute cerebral hemorrhage, especially many patients with sub-arachnoid hemorrhage, will present with only a severe and unusual headache. These patients are neurologically intact, which means that their neurological examination is normal. There is no facial droop, no arm weakness, no dragging of the leg. They speak normally and understand normally. They just have a very bad and abrupt onset of headache. This was how Sharon Stone presented and was part of the reason that she waited for several days before going to the hospital.

As a general rule, sudden onset of one or more of the following symptoms should be considered to be caused by a stroke until a reasonable evaluation by a physician concludes otherwise: numbness of the face, arm, or leg, especially if on one side of the body; problems with vision in one or both eyes; confusion, problems speaking or understanding; difficulty walking, severe vertigo, loss of balance or coordination; and severe and unusual headache.

We will also discuss the concept of stroke units more in subsequent chapters, but a few words are necessary here as well. That is because the ambulance crew has to decide where to take a patient with a possible stroke. Now that we have more effective but time-dependent treatments, the paramedics and EMTs have an important decision to make. That is why the various pre-hospital stroke scales were developed: to help paramedics decide which patients are having strokes and which are not.

The concept of bypassing a closer hospital for one that is farther away is not a new one. The best example in the United States relates to trauma care. A patient in a serious automobile crash may be transported to a hospital farther away that has more resources available, although there is a much closer one to the site of the crash. The concept is that the greater resources (doctors, nurses, operating rooms, specialists, and special equipment) available at the farther site more than make up for the additional transport time. This is well accepted for trauma care, and there is a movement to begin doing similar pre-hospital triage for heart attack patients.

This same concept is working its way into stroke care with the development of stroke centers. We will discuss these centers in far greater detail in Chapters 4 and 5, but for now, consider that rapid transport to a hospital that has all the various resources for diagnosis and treatment of stroke patients is very important, and there is a balance between rapid care and the best care.

4

Diagnosis of Stroke

When any physician sees any patient, the physician uses a process of simple logic to try to sort out what the cause of a patient's symptoms is. Doctors use this same process whether a patient complains of left-sided weakness, a sore throat, or chest pain. For example, when a doctor sees a patient with a sore throat, many possibilities exist. It could be strep (caused by the streptococcus bacterium), but it also could be mononucleosis or some other virus causing the sore throat. Less likely possibilities include inflammation of the thyroid gland or a foreign body, say a fish bone, that became stuck. An immigrant who comes to an ED with a sore throat and who may not be fully immunized could even have diphtheria as a cause of their symptoms.

The doctor uses various tools such as the patient's history and a physical examination before then deciding what tests to order. If he thinks strep is a good possibility, the doctor might order a strep culture to confirm his clinical suspicion, or if he is pretty certain, he may simply start an antibiotic such as penicillin to begin treating without any further diagnostic testing.

The term for this general process is "differential diagnosis." What is happening in the doctor's mind is that he makes a list of all the possible causes of a given patient's symptoms and then, by answers to questions or findings on the physical examination and results of tests, decides which possibilities to take off the list and which to keep on. In the first minutes of the evaluation, the emergency physician is going through a process of trying to sort out exactly what is the cause of the patient's symptoms.

When a stroke patient arrives at the ED, especially if they arrive within several hours of onset of symptoms, the clock is ticking. The physicians and nurses must perform this differential diagnostic process very rapidly. The problem is that patients do not roll into the ED with a sign on their forehead that says "stroke patient"; they arrive with various symptoms that usually (but not always) include some kind of focal weakness.

Therefore, the first step is to verify that this particular patient is in fact having a stroke and not some other condition that can mimic a stroke. In some cases, this is very easy to do, but in other cases, it can be quite difficult. Table 4.1 lists some of the conditions that can masquerade as a stroke. The nurses and physicians must quickly but methodically go through this process of ruling out other conditions and trying to rule in a stroke.

This process begins to occur even before the patient comes to the ED if they arrive by ambulance. The paramedics will have already begun to consider other possible causes of the acute onset of neurological symptoms. One simple test that the paramedics in the ambulance will always do is to check the patient's blood sugar. Current technology allows the paramedics in the field, or nurses in the ED, to prick the patient's finger and then place a drop of blood onto a strip of paper. This strip is inserted into a tiny device that measures blood sugar, similar to the devices that diabetic people use in their homes. These devices give a very precise level of the glucose in the bloodstream.

The reason this is so important is that patients with low blood sugar, called hypoglycemia, can have symptoms that can look exactly like a stroke. Most patients with hypoglycemia will have more generalized symptoms (sweating,

Table 4.1.
Stroke Mimics

Low blood sugar (hypoglycemia)
Postseizure weakness (Todd's paralysis)
Migraine
TIA
Brain tumor
Other mass lesions such as brain abscess
Multiple sclerosis
Subdural (or epidural) bleeding
Unmasking an old stroke

palpitations, confusion, or fuzzy thinking) and not the more focal ones typical of a stroke. However, some patients with a low blood sugar will have specific focal symptoms, such as a droopy face on one side and weakness of the same-side arm. If the low blood sugar is recognized and treated with intravenous or oral sugar, these symptoms will vanish within minutes. Also, a high blood sugar reading has significance if the patient is having a stroke, because high levels may lead to worse outcomes in stroke patients, and these levels can be lowered with insulin. Other metabolic problems such as a very low or very high sodium level in the blood can sometimes produce the same effects.

Another common problem is a patient who has had a seizure. After a seizure, most patients are temporarily confused, and some patients will have focal weakness as well. These symptoms can last for minutes to hours. If a patient has a seizure, especially if the seizure was not recognized by the people who called the paramedics, then the medical personnel may only see a confused patient with focal weakness. This situation is called "Todd's paralysis" and it is perfectly compatible with a stroke. Once again, it shows how important the patient's history is to help guide the physician to start the right therapy.

Migraine is present in approximately 12 percent of the general population and is among the most common causes of headache known. Some patients with migraine will suffer from periods of focal weakness, which are almost always temporary. Although this happens in a very small percentage of migraine patients, migraine is so common that even a small percentage of a very large number is significant. There is no specific test to rule out a migraine, and usually these attacks occur in patients with a past history of migraine and similar episodes. However, in the occasional patient whose first migraine presents in this manner or someone whose previous migraines did not manifest this kind of symptom, a physician may well diagnose a stroke.

We talked earlier about TIA; obviously in the first minutes to hours of a TIA, a physician could not accurately make the distinction between these two entities. This distinction may not even be important because, for the most part, TIA and stroke are really two different parts of the same disease and are treated in many ways just like a stroke.

Patients with brain tumors usually present to their physician with a history of slow, gradual onset of whatever symptoms their tumor produces. In some patients, these symptoms may be headache with vomiting or double vision, but they can also include focal weakness. In the typical brain tumor case in which the symptoms develop very slowly, it is quite clear that such a patient is not having a stroke. However, occasionally, a brain tumor patient can present with symptoms that are much more abrupt. This is possible if a tumor has been causing a gradual increase in pressure on a given area of brain, which at

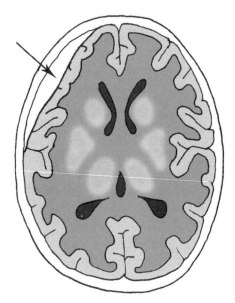

Figure 4.1. A subdural hematoma (arrow) that is external to the brain and that is pushing on the brain. This bleeding is usually caused by head trauma that breaks blood vessels near the surface of the brain. Sometimes a subdural hematoma can mimic a stroke, especially in older patients.

some critical point causes enough pressure to start causing symptoms. Once again, in this situation, a tumor could be confused with a stroke.

The same thing can happen with a subdural hematoma (see Figure 4.1). A bit more background information about brain anatomy is necessary here. You have probably heard the term "meningitis," which means an inflammation (usually caused by an infection) of the meninges. The meninges are the protective covering of the brain, and there are three layers (see Figure 4.2). The outermost is a tough membrane called the dura. Beneath the dura is a spidery web-like membrane called the arachnoid. It is below this membrane where subarachnoid hemorrhages (like the one Sharon Stone suffered) occur. Beneath the arachnoid is the very thin "pia," which is tightly adhered to the actual brain. Patients with subdural hemorrhage have bleeding beneath the dura (but outside of the arachnoid).

This bleeding is almost always caused by a broken blood vessel, usually a vein, so most patients with subdural hematoma will have a history of trauma. Some will have an abrupt onset of symptoms. However, in some patients, there is no history of trauma, because either the injury was very minor or it was days to weeks ago and the patient simply does not recall it. This group of

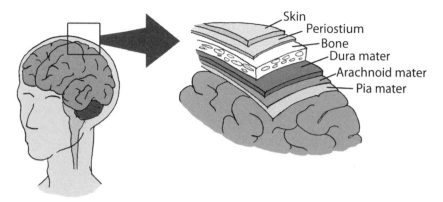

Figure 4.2. The relationship of the three layers of the meninges (dura, arachnoid, and pia) to the scalp and skull on the outside and to the brain on the inside. The meninges help to protect the brain. The subarachnoid space is between the arachnoid and the pia. When a person has meningitis, they have an infection of the meninges.

patients may suddenly become aware of their symptoms (although the bleeding has developed slowly). This actually happens relatively frequently, especially in the elderly who are at higher risk of stroke as well.

Yet another possibility is that a patient has had a minor stroke in the past but does not have a permanent neurological deficit. That is to say, they are functionally normal on a day-to-day basis. However, some interval medical problem (such as pneumonia, a urinary tract infection, or mild congestive heart failure) can alter their normal balance. This physiologic alteration can "unmask" the old stroke. To the clinicians in the ED, this patient could appear exactly how a patient with a new stroke would appear.

With this background in mind, one can see how medical personnel use the process of differential diagnosis in stroke patients. So the first step of diagnosis is the history. There are many components that are important within the history. Because the patient may have an altered mental status or have an inability to express themselves as a result of aphasia, the doctors and nurses must often gather their information from family members, shopkeepers, coworkers, or other eyewitnesses and, of course, the paramedics and EMTs who have dealt with that patient.

Because strokes are more important in older patients, the person's age is of obvious significance. The paramedics, nurses, and doctors will all try to piece together what the specific symptoms are, precisely when they started, how they evolved, what the patient was doing at the onset, and all of the other relevant details of the event. Essentially, they are trying to exactly recreate the sequence of events.

Seemingly minor details can be very important in this part of the history. For example, did the patient go to sleep normal and then wake up with right-sided weakness? If so, how long did they sleep? Did the left-sided facial droop precede the left arm weakness by thirty minutes or did both start together? Has this patient with a migraine headache ever had double vision with a previous migraine or not? In fleshing out the story here, the doctor is acting like a detective, trying to get all the facts to sort out which are relevant and which are not. In many ways, this process of differential diagnosis is much like a policeman trying to solve a crime.

Doctors will ask about associated symptoms. For example, the presence of fever suggests the possibility of a heart infection called endocarditis that might have caused an embolism to the brain. The fever also alerts the clinician that perhaps this is some sort of infection that is unmasking an old stroke. Any associated symptoms could be significant. Shortness of breath might indicate heart failure or pneumonia. Neck pain could indicate a dissection of one of the arteries that lead into the Circle of Willis. Vomiting, double vision, or vertigo suggests a stroke in the cerebellum or brainstem. A severe headache could indicate a subarachnoid hemorrhage, among other possibilities.

Asking about past history and what medications the patient is taking can be important. This part of the history is essential in identifying risk factors (see Chapter 2). Does the patient have a past history of heart attack or atrial fibrillation? Have they had a TIA in the recent past? Have they ever used illicit drugs such as "speed" or cocaine (which can lead to blood vessel problems in the brain)? Do they have any known problems with blood clotting or are they taking medications that artificially thin the blood (making bleeding more likely)?

All of this information is assembled as rapidly as possible, often within minutes. Next, the physician assesses the patient's neurological status. To some extent, this begins simultaneously with taking the history as the doctor looks for any facial asymmetry, slurred speech, or other abnormalities that may be evident from just looking at and talking to another person. The general appearance of a patient is an important portion of the physical examination. As well, the doctor will look at the vital signs as they are either recorded on the chart or appear on the monitor at the head of the patient's bed.

The vital signs include the temperature, pulse rate, blood pressure, and respiratory rate. Increasingly, some include the oxygen level as the "fifth" vital sign. Abnormalities in any of these can be very useful for the physician, not only in diagnosing a stroke but in taking care of the all-important "ABCs" of patient care: airway, breathing, and circulation. For example, if the patient is not breathing properly or is not getting enough oxygen, or if a dangerously high pulse or low blood pressure exists, the doctor will need to stabilize this life-threatening situation even before taking the history. For the present discussion, let us assume that there are no life-threatening vital signs (we will discuss these in more details in Chapter 5).

Abnormal vital signs can suggest various causes of a patient's stroke. For example, an irregular pulse suggests atrial fibrillation that could be the reason that a patient has an embolism that has lodged in the brain. This is one reason that all stroke patients have an electrocardiogram (ECG) done. This is a simple test whereby electrodes are placed on a patient's limbs and chest and the electrical output from the heart is measured. This electrical output is printed onto a piece of paper that is then interpreted by the physician. Very high blood pressure could be attributable to the brain's reaction to diminished blood flow, in an attempt to keep the flow of nutrients available in the area of decrease. As mentioned before, fever can be a sign of a bloodstream or heart infection causing a stroke, and a low oxygen level shows that supplemental oxygen must be given.

The remainder of the physical examination is traditionally divided into the "general" exam (all organs except for the nervous system) and the neurological system (see Table 4.2). The general exam may show a murmur in the neck from a partially blocked carotid artery. Another possibility is a heart murmur that could be a clue of an embolism from the heart to the brain. However, the most important part of the physical examination here is the neurological exam.

The traditional neurological examination is in several parts: mental status; cranial nerves; motor exam; sensory exam; cerebellar exam; gait (how the

Table 4.2.
Diagnostic Tests for Stroke Patients (not all are performed initially)

In all patients
    Blood tests: blood count, serum glucose and chemistries, kidney function, clotting tests
    ECG
    Brain imaging, usually CT scan or MRI
    Telemetry to monitor for arrhythmias
    Carotid ultrasound (or other test for carotid artery blockage)
In some patients
    Cerebrovascular imaging
    Chest x-ray
    Echocardiogram
    Lumbar puncture
    Urinalysis

patient walks); and reflexes. Although all of these are important, the first three are more important in the majority of stroke patients. There are various stroke scales or stroke scoring systems that physicians in the hospital use, and the most important is the National Institutes of Health Stroke Scale (NIHSS). This is an eleven-part, forty-two-point scale that allows the neurological examination to be quantified and compared from one patient to another (for research) and within one patient at one point in time versus another (to measure improvement). It is certainly not necessary to learn or know the NIHSS unless you are a clinician caring for stroke patients, but, for interested readers, it is duplicated in Table 4.3. In essence, the NIHSS is a very regimented neurological examination that assigns a number at the end of the exam. Different components measure neurological function in all parts of the brain, including mental status, vision, reading, speaking and comprehension, and strength and sensation.

After the history and physical examination have been done and the basic laboratory tests and ECG are obtained, the clinician will do some kind of brain imaging. It is important to know that, although the lab tests are sent off, the doctor does not wait for the results before proceeding with the brain imaging.

There are many types of brain imaging, but the most commonly performed one is the CT scan. This test is a form of x-ray that first became clinically available in the early 1970s. The patient lies on a special stretcher called a gantry. Once the patient is lying down, the gantry is slid into a large round cylinder that slowly spins around the patient to obtain images from 360 degrees. Then a computer, using sophisticated software, generates the images of the brain. The Latin root "tomo" means a cut or a slice. The computer software makes a picture of various slices of the brain. Figure 4.3 shows a typical "slice" in the middle of the head.

The first generation of CT scanners took about thirty to forty-five minutes just to image the brain. Currently available scanners take about ten seconds and collect pictures that are far clearer than those that were available with older scanners. This time factor is important. If a patient moves inside the scanner, the quality of the images is poor, just like if one were taking a photograph of a moving target. The images are blurred. With the faster machines, even a patient who is somewhat uncooperative in the machine can have crisp, clear images obtained.

Nearly every ED in the United States has a CT scanner available. For the most part, these machines are located very close to the ED; in fact, it takes more time to wheel the patient to the machine and transfer them from their stretcher to the gantry than to actually obtain the CT scan images. The

Table 4.3.
NIH Stroke Scale

1A. Level of consciousness (LOC): test of LOC, ranging from alert to comatose

0	Alert: patient is fully alert and keenly responsive
1	Drowsy: patient is drowsy but can be aroused with minor stimulation; the patient obeys, answers, and responds to commands
2	Stuporous: patient is lethargic but requires repeated stimulation to attend; the patient may need painful or strong stimuli to respond to or follow commands
3	Coma: patient is comatose and responds only with reflexive motor or automatic responses; otherwise, the patient is unresponsive

1B. LOC questions. The doctors asks the patient two questions: "What is the month of the year?" and "How old are you?"

0	Answers both correctly
1	Answers one correctly
2	Both incorrect

1C. LOC commands: The doctor asks the patient to follow two commands: open and close his/her eyes and then is asked to make a grip (close and open his/her hand).

0	Obeys both correctly
1	Obeys one correctly
2	Both incorrect

2. Gaze (ability of eyes to move across the midline): The doctor simply asks the patient to look all the way to the left and then all the way to the right to test the ability of the eyes to track to both sides.

0	Normal: the patient has normal lateral eye movements
1	Partial gaze palsy: the patient is unable to move one or both eyes completely to both directions
2	Forced deviation: the patient has conjugate deviation of the eyes to the right or left, even with reflexive movements

3. Visual fields: The doctor tests to see whether the patient can see to both sides. The word "hemianopia" means a loss of sight to one half of the visual field. The term "quadrantic field defect" refers to loss of sight to a quarter of the visual field. Think of half a pizza or a quarter of a pizza.

0	No visual loss
1	Partial hemianopia: there is a partial visual field defect in both eyes; included is a quadrantic field defect or sector field defect
2	Complete hemianopia: there is dense visual field defect in both eyes
3	Bilateral hemianopia: there are bilateral visual field defects in both eyes. Cortical blindness is included

4. Facial movement (facial weakness): The doctor assesses how symmetric the face is. Sometimes the patient will be asked to grimace or smile or puff out their cheeks to test for facial weakness.

0	Normal facial movements; no asymmetry.
1	Minor paresis: asymmetrical facial movements or facial asymmetry at rest; this response may be noted with a spontaneous smile but not with forced facial movements

(continued)

Table 4.3.
(Continued)

| 2 | Partial paresis, unilateral "central" facial paresis: decreased spontaneous and forced facial movements with changes most prominent at the mouth; orbital and forehead musculature movements are normal |
| 3 | Complete palsy: dysfunction involves forehead, orbital, and circumoral muscles (the entire distribution of the facial nerve); deficits may be unilateral or bilateral (facial diplegia) complete facial paresis |

5. Motor function of arms (left and right): The clinician asks the patient to hold out the arms forward with the palms facing the ceiling, "as if you were holding up a tray," for 10 seconds duration.

0	No drift: the patient is able to hold the outstretched limb for 10 seconds
1	Drift: the patient is able to hold the outstretched limb for 10 seconds but there is some fluttering or drift of the limb; if the limb falls to an intermediate position, the score is 1
2	Some effort against gravity: the patient is not able to hold the outstretched limb for 10 seconds but there is some effort against gravity
3	No effort against gravity: the patient is not able to bring the limb off the bed but there is some effort against gravity; if the limb is raised in the correct position by the examiner, the patient is unable to sustain the position
4	No movement: the patient is unable to move the limb; there is no effort against gravity
9	Untestable: may be used only if the limb is missing or amputated or if the shoulder joint is fused

6. Motor function of legs (right and left): Similar to the arm motor function test; the patient is asked to hold the outstretched leg 30 degrees above the bed for 5 seconds.

0	No drift: the patient is able to hold the outstretched limb for 5 seconds
1	Drift: the patient is able to hold the outstretched limb for 5 seconds, but there is unsteadiness, fluttering, or drift of the limb
2	Some effort against gravity: the patient is unable to hold the outstretched limb for 5 seconds but there is some effort against gravity
3	No effort against gravity: the patient is not able to bring the limb off the bed but there is effort against gravity. If the limb is placed in the correct position, the patient is unable to sustain the position
4	No movement: the patient is unable to move the limb; there is no effort against gravity
9	Untestable: may be used only if limb is missing or hip joint is fused

7. Limb ataxia: This item is aimed at examining the patient for evidence of a unilateral cerebellar lesion. Ataxia means clumsiness and decreased accuracy of limb movement.

0	Absent: the patient is able to perform both the finger-to nose and heel-to-shin tasks well; the movements are smooth and accurate
1	Present unilaterally in either arm or leg; the patient is able to perform one of the two required tasks well
2	Present unilaterally in both arm and leg or bilaterally: the patient is unable to perform either task well. Movements are inaccurate, clumsy, or poorly done

(continued)

Table 4.3.
(Continued)

9	Untestable: may be used only if all Motor function scores = 4, limb is missing, amputated, or fused, or if item 1A.LOC = 3

8. Sensory: The doctor touches all four limbs of the patient with a paper clip, or gently with a pin, to test for presence of sensation.

0   Normal: no sensory loss to pin is detected

1   Partial loss: mild to moderate diminution in perception to pin stimulation is recognized; this may involve more than one limb

2   Dense loss: severe sensory loss so that the patient is not aware of being touched; patient does not respond to noxious stimuli applied to that side of the body

9. Best language: the patient is presented with three standard sentences and asked to read them. The response shows how well they can read the text.

0   No aphasia: the patient is able to read the sentences well and is able to correctly name the objects on the sheet of paper

1   Mild to moderate aphasia: the patient has mild to moderate naming errors, word finding errors, paraphasias, or mild impairment in comprehension or expression

2   Severe aphasia: the patient has severe aphasia with difficulty in reading as well as naming objects. Patient with either Broca's or Wernicke's aphasia is included here

3   Mute

10. Dysarthria: In this component of the NIHSS, the patient's ability to articulate given words is tested. Again, the physician presents a card with standard words and asks the patient to read them.

0   Normal articulation: patient is able to pronounce the words clearly and without any problem in articulation

1   Mild to moderate dysarthria: patient has problems in articulation; mild to moderate slurring of words is noted; the patient can be understood but with some difficulty

3   Near unintelligible or worse: patient's speech is so slurred that it is unintelligible

9   Untestable: may be used only if item 9, Best language = 3, or if the patient has an endotracheal tube

11. Neglect (extinction and inattention): The terms "extinction" and "inattention" have to do with the brain's ability to take in events or images from both sides of the body. In this test, patients are shown a standard picture with actions occurring on both the right and the left. They are asked "what do you see in this picture?"

0   No neglect: the patient is able to recognize bilateral simultaneous cutaneous stimuli on the right and left sides of the body and is able to identify images on the right and left sides of the picture

1   Partial neglect: the patient is able to recognize either cutaneous or visual stimuli on both the left and right, but is unable to do both successfully (unless severe visual loss or aphasia is present)

2   Complete neglect: the patient is unable to recognize either bilateral cutaneous sensory or visual stimuli

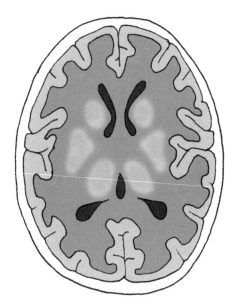

Figure 4.3. A normal brain "slice" about halfway down. Notice that there are folds of brain (called sulci) all around the outside. These are lost sometimes in stroke (see Figures 4.4 and 4.5) and in subdural hematoma (see Figure 4.1). The areas represented in black are the fluid (CSF)-filled ventricles. When intracranial pressure is high, these ventricles will be pushed closed.

images, which are for the most part digitized as of the year 2008, are instantly available for interpretation, to both the clinicians and the radiologists.

There are several reasons to have a CT scan done. First of all, some patients will show a diagnosis other than stroke. For example, a brain abscess or tumor or a subdural hematoma may show up on the scan. In this case, an alternative diagnosis (one of the stroke mimics) will be apparent. Second, in the case of stroke, the CT scan is an excellent way to discriminate between an ischemic and a hemorrhagic stroke. In an acute, or fresh, hemorrhagic stroke, the blood will appear bright white (see Figure 4.4). In patients with ischemic stroke, the CT findings will depend on how old the stroke is. In very acute situations, say the first six to twelve hours, the CT scan may be completely normal. Over time, however, the brain in the area of an ischemic stroke will become blacker than the surrounding tissue (see Figure 4.5).

The CT scan can be done within minutes of arrival to the ED and, by AHA guidelines, is supposed to be done within twenty minutes of arrival. This scan is vitally important for early-presenting patients because its results will drive the decision making about treatment (more about this in Chapter 6).

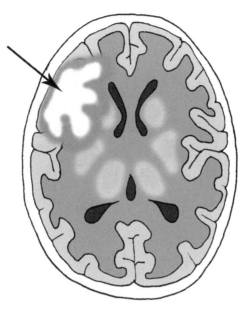

Figure 4.4. Illustration of a hemorrhagic stroke (arrow). Acute blood appears white on the CT scan and is usually easy to see on the CT. Distinguishing an ischemic stroke from a hemorrhagic one is very important, as we will see in later chapters. Fortunately, it is usually easy to see the difference.

Sometimes, in larger hospitals that have the ability to perform a rapid magnetic resonance imaging (MRI) scan, this is done in place of the CT scan. The MRI is a totally different way of looking at the brain (or other tissues in the body). All x-rays (including CT scans) use ionizing radiation to distinguish between different densities of tissue. The MRI uses magnetic fields to help distinguish between these densities, so it shows different kinds of distinctions than does the CT. In general, an MRI scan of a given body part takes longer to obtain the images, is less commonly available on an emergency basis, and is more expensive. At the same time, the MRI gives images that far better distinguish between various tissues and show changes much sooner (after symptom onset) than a CT scan.

For example, although it takes many hours for a CT to show an acute ischemic stroke, the MRI will begin to show changes within minutes! Also, as MRI technology has improved, its ability to distinguish between hemorrhage and ischemia (as well as the various stroke mimics) is as good as, if not better than, CT. If MRI were as quick and easy and available as CT, it would clearly be the superior test. However, the current state of diagnostics is such that CT is the test that is most commonly performed in the ED. Later in their hospital

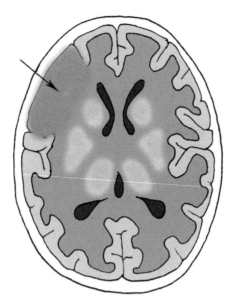

Figure 4.5. An acute ischemic stroke in the early hours (arrow). Note the loss of the normal sulci, but the color on the CT is often the same as the normal uninvolved brain. Notice that there is no signs of elevated pressure (the black ventricles are preserved in size and shape).

stay, many of these patients will have follow-up MRI scans to better delineate the precise nature of that patient's stroke. Figure 4.6 shows MRI images of a patient with an acute ischemic stroke.

Both CT and MRI can also image the blood vessels that feed the brain. These are called CT angiography (CTA) and MR angiography (MRA). This is the other diagnostic imaging test that is sometimes done acutely. There is a balance between the doctor's desire to know as much as possible about a particular patient's stroke and the need to obtain information as rapidly as possible. A physician who has more knowledge about the kind of stroke that a given patient has can administer a more rational treatment to that patient. For this reason, doctors will usually do vascular imaging tests such as CTA or MRA to try to pinpoint the vascular lesion that has caused the stroke.

One can imagine that a patient who has a middle cerebral artery stroke that is incomplete and who has a persistently blocked middle cerebral artery might respond better to a treatment designed to open the artery than another patient whose stroke is complete and whose artery is open. These tests of vascular imaging are not routinely done, and, in fact, in smaller hospitals (where most stroke care is currently delivered), they are not standard.

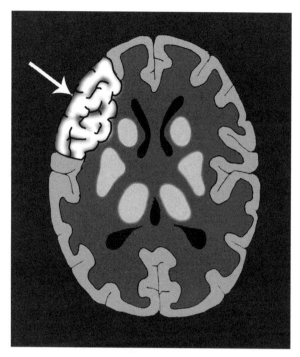

Figure 4.6. Illustration of how an ischemic stroke appears (arrow) on an MRI scan. You can see that the area of stroke is much clearer than on a CT, and the underlying structures are more apparent. MRI allows much better diagnosis than CT, but MRI is more expensive, less available, and takes much longer to accomplish than CT. Over time, MRI will likely become the standard, but this may take many years.

All of these tests have three objectives. First, the doctor wants to exclude stroke mimics. Second, the doctor wants to define what subtype of stroke is occurring. Last, the doctor wants to gather information that will help define the best treatment.

There are other diagnostics that are done in the hospital but after the initial emergency care. Those will be discussed in Chapter 10 because they have more to do with preventing complications and improving long-term outcomes.

There are two other concepts that impact the diagnosis of stroke patients. The first is that of a "stroke team." This is another concept borrowed from trauma care. In larger hospitals, when a severely traumatized patient arrives in the ED, for example after a severe car crash, a team of physicians, nurses, and other healthcare providers collect and work collaboratively to rapidly assess and treat the patient. This same concept is now being applied to stroke victims. In larger hospitals, personnel from the ED, neurologists, radiologists, and laboratory technicians will all be notified at the same time, sometimes by the EMTs even before the patient has arrived.

Everyone has a preassigned role. This method of care speeds the evaluation, getting the CT scan, interpreting the CT scan, getting the results of the laboratory tests and the ECG, starting the cardiac monitoring, etc. This has become an important concept because some of the treatments for stroke are very time dependent, some necessary within three hours of onset of symptoms.

The last concept in the diagnosis of stroke is that of "telemedicine." In most hospitals across the country, there is no neurologist immediately available in the ED. One may be on-call by telephone, but decisions must be made very quickly and this does not allow enough time for them to come to the hospital from home. As well, some emergency physicians may want consultation with a neurologist before using some of the more powerful stroke treatments (for more details, see Chapter 6). Therefore, the concept of having stroke specialists available to "examine" the patient from a remote location has been used, and this is called telemedicine.

Using a webcam pointed at the patient, the remote stroke specialist can actually do the NIHSS on a patient and see the results. Because the CT scan can be digitized and also examined remotely, the stroke specialist can have all the relevant information to help the on-site emergency physician make the best decision as to what kind of therapy should be given. The next three chapters will describe the various treatments used for different kinds of stroke.

5

General Treatment of Stroke

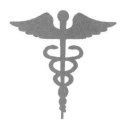

I n Chapters 6 and 7, we will discuss specific treatments of ischemic stroke and hemorrhagic stroke. However, there are many elements in stroke therapy that are common to both types, and we will discuss them in this chapter.

ABCs

As mentioned earlier, in the treatment of any patient, with any problem, the first things that a physician addresses are the so-called ABCs. If these most basic bodily processes are not functioning, then anything else done to the patient is meaningless. Even the most sophisticated stroke treatments performed in the best stroke unit in the world by the most knowledgeable neurologists would be pointless if the patient is not breathing or has no pulse.

A is for airway. This can be an important issue for stroke patients. For example, if a person having a stroke has a decreased level of consciousness, their tongue may fall back in the throat and lead to upper airway obstruction. Upper airway obstruction will be rapidly fatal if it is complete and if it is not treated immediately. Sometimes, all that is needed is to reposition the jaw, pulling it forward as is taught in cardiopulmonary resuscitation training, or the situation may be as simple as a patient's dentures have fallen out of place and are obstructing the airway. Simply removing the dentures may be all that is needed to remedy this situation. Other times, all that may be required is to suction out some respiratory secretions that are blocking the flow of air.

Other situations require other solutions. In some patients, a flexible rubber tube can be inserted into the nose and then slid into the upper airway to open this passage. This may be necessary to maintain a space between that floppy tongue and the back of the throat. In a worst-case situation, if a stroke patient is not breathing at all or is breathing inadequately, the physician or paramedic must insert a flexible silicon breathing tube into the mouth and then direct it into the trachea (windpipe). This is not very commonly needed in stroke patients. However, endotracheal intubation is more commonly needed in hemorrhagic strokes (rather than in ischemic ones) and with posterior circulation strokes (rather than with anterior ones). The important concept is that, if the airway is not working properly, all other efforts will be futile.

B is for breathing. Once the airway is established and secure, breathing must be ensured. Again, for most stroke patients, this is not an issue, although for some it may be. For example, because most stroke patients are older, they often have other simultaneous medical conditions; if some involve the lung (severe obstructive lung disease or a resolving pneumonia), then they may need assistance with their breathing. Another possibility is that they may be taking various medications that are sedating. Too much sedation can also decrease a patient's ability to adequately breathe. The question arises: does the patient require supplemental oxygen? Most stroke patients do not; however, for patients whose oxygen levels are low, the clinician will need to administer supplemental oxygen via a mask or small nasal prongs that are connected to an oxygen source. A patient's oxygen level can be easily measured by a simple instrument that looks like a clothespin; it is placed on the patient's fingertip and will continuously read out the person's oxygen level. Some researchers have even experimented with hyperbaric oxygen (pressurized oxygen that can increase oxygen delivery to the tissues), but this modality, although theoretically appealing, has not been proven to be beneficial.

C is for circulation, which means, is there sufficient blood flow? We have already learned that, by definition of a stroke, there is not sufficient blood flow to the affected areas of the brain. In the context of ABCs, the circulation refers to the general circulation; is the blood pressure high enough? Is it too high?

BLOOD PRESSURE CONTROL

Something that is seemingly so simple and basic is actually fraught with a great deal of controversy. One general principle with respect to blood pressure in the setting of acute stroke is certain; neither a blood pressure that is too high nor too low is good for stroke patients. The wise physician will consider the ideal blood flow to the brain for an individual patient and not just derive a "one size fits all" approach. No one target pressure will work for all patients. Although official recommendations are a bit different for different kinds of strokes, we will discuss the topic of blood pressure treatment in all types of stroke here.

Four physiological terms are important to understand this: mean arterial blood pressure (MAP), cerebral perfusion pressure (CPP), ICP, and cerebral blood flow (CBF).

No matter what the stroke type or whether the blood pressure is thought to be too high or too low, the guiding concepts relate to the CPP and the CBF. These two variables are related, but they are not the same thing. To best understand this section on blood pressure, the reader is encouraged to read these next several paragraphs; however, if this aspect of stroke care is not relevant to your specific research project, you can pick up at the next heading, Guidelines for Elevated Blood Pressure.

Normally we report the blood pressure as two numbers: the upper (systolic) over the lower (diastolic). So a normal blood pressure might be 120 over 80 (120/80). The actual unit of pressure used is millimeters of mercury, but for simplicity, we'll leave that off. The upper number is the pressure measured in an artery at the height of the heart contraction (called systole) and the lower number is measured when the heart is at relaxation (called diastole). Physiologists often use the term MAP to account for the average pressure in the arteries during a cardiac cycle. The usual formula that is used for this is as follows: MAP = diastolic pressure + $\frac{1}{3}$ (systolic – diastolic). So in the case of 120/80, the MAP would be 93 (80 + $\frac{1}{3}$ of 40 [120 – 80]). This MAP is the pressure that drives blood through the brain.

However, there is resistance to this as well. The contents of the skull (the brain, the CSF, and the blood itself) also exert some pressure, the ICP. This pressure gives some resistance to the MAP pushing the blood in. This is because the blood vessels are not rigid pipes but muscular, flexible tubes. So any pressure on their outside will lead to resistance to flow on the inside. Imagine a glass fishbowl full of jelly. This jelly would exert a given pressure against the inside of the bowl. Now imagine a series of elastic tubes that pump fluid into one side of the bowl, through it, and then out the other side. The force that "drives" this fluid through the tube and out the other side is the perfusion pressure. It equals the pressure of the fluid pushing on the inside of the tube minus the pressure of the jelly pushing against the outside of the tube. In the case of the brain, it equals the blood pressure minus the ICP. Therefore, the CPP = MAP – ICP (see Figure 5.1).

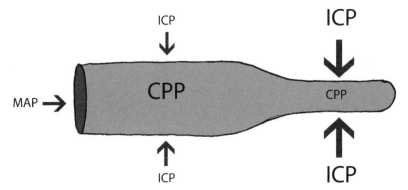

Figure 5.1. Illustration of how the blood pressure flowing into a blood vessel (MAP) is reduced by whatever ambient ICP exists. The difference is the CPP. As ICP increases, the CPP decreases for a given level of blood pressure.

The other half of the concept is that of CBF. This is different from CPP and more important. Pressure is critical because it supports flow to the brain tissue. It is the flow of oxygen-rich and glucose-rich blood that is important. Millions of years of evolution have made the brain remarkably resourceful, and so its blood vessels will often make these adjustments automatically. If it senses that it is not receiving enough blood flow (either because of decreased CPP or increased ICP), it will alter one of those variables to keep the CBF constant. This process is called "autoregulation." Autoregulation attempts to maintain a constant blood flow to the brain across wide ranges of blood pressure (see Figure 5.2).

To see how this works in practice, let's first discuss the situation of the blood pressure being too low. The first thing the doctor will consider is why it is low. Is the patient dehydrated because they have been vomiting or have not been taking enough fluids in the preceding hours? Is it low because the patient is taking powerful medications to lower their blood pressure as treatment for their hypertension? Or have they had a heart attack that has left their heart muscle incapable of pumping enough blood to mount a normal blood pressure? Is their heart rhythm abnormal and to blame? Is this a young patient whose normal blood pressure is simply lower than the average stroke patient? Each of these possibilities needs to be rapidly considered because the treatment may be different for each of them.

Each cause may lead to a different solution; however, all of these causes may relate to a low CPP. All of the interventions that a physician may try are guided by the simple formula: CPP = MAP − ICP. If the blood pressure is too

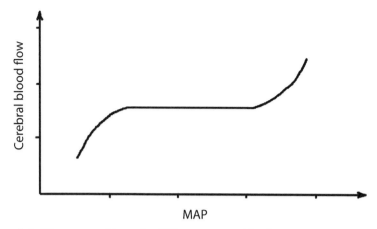

Figure 5.2. Illustration of how the CBF is constant (the flat portion of the curve in the middle) over wide ranges of MAP. It also shows that, when the blood pressure falls too low (left side of graph), autoregulation fails and the CBF flow plummets. Similarly, on the right side of the graph, if the MAP is too high, autoregulation will also fail and the CBF can become dangerously high.

low, then the CPP will be too low and must be raised. In this situation, doctors will give intravenous medications that pharmacologically raise the blood pressure, which in turn will improve the CPP. This in turn will improve CBF, but this may be especially beneficial to the area of the brain affected by the stroke.

The possibility of cardiac pumping problems or an abnormal heart rhythm (either causing low blood pressure) are two reasons that all stroke patients are placed on a cardiac monitor, so that these parameters can be continuously measured. As well, all these patients have ECGs performed to look for signs of heart attack, abnormal heart rhythms, or other cardiac problems that might be relevant to their care.

The approach to an elevated blood pressure, hypertension, is much more complicated. This is because both the MAP and the ICP can change over time. For example, patients with chronic hypertension, a very common condition in stroke patients, may require a higher blood pressure to perfuse their brains. This is because, over years of this condition, their arteries become more rigid and less elastic. In this case, they require a higher MAP to maintain CBF at a given level. Furthermore, when a patient has a stroke, the involved portion of the brain often swells. Because this swelling takes place in the skull, a rigid box, the ICP goes up. Therefore, for the CPP to remain constant, the MAP needs to go up, too, to overcome the increased resistance of the higher ICP. This is when autoregulation kicks in. It is important to know, however, that this process has its limits. Some blood pressures are either too high or too low for the body to "autoregulate" its own way out of it.

The doctor can measure the blood pressure easily, just like when you are in his office. However, CPP and CBF cannot be so easily measured, nor can ICP. Just like solving any algebraic equation with three variables, you need to know two of the three to calculate the third. Measuring the ICP is relatively easy, but it involves an invasive surgical procedure (drilling a very small hole into the skull through which a pressure gauge is inserted). If the doctor knew the ICP and the BP, then he would know what the CPP was and know exactly what variable to manipulate. Generally, we do not measure the ICP in stroke patients, at least those outside of the intensive care unit (ICU). So the doctor will try to estimate the ICP by using the neurological examination.

GUIDELINES FOR ELEVATED BLOOD PRESSURE

All that said, most official guidelines, such as those by the AHA, tend to err on the side of letting the blood pressure trend higher during a stroke so as to allow the process of autoregulation a chance to maximize CBF. At extremely high levels, however, doctors will administer various medications to lower the blood pressure. Generally, doctors use lower target blood pressures for patients with hemorrhagic strokes than they do for ischemic strokes. For the most part, they will use intravenous medications that can be increased or decreased quickly and whose effects will rapidly follow. As a general rule, if a patient with an ischemic stroke's blood pressure is greater than 185/110, then doctors will usually treat that patient with blood-pressure-lowering medications. It is important to know, however, that without knowing the ICP and calculating the CPP and CBF, these target numbers are somewhat arbitrary. Different targets may be best for different individuals.

TEMPERATURE

We learned earlier that fever can be a sign of an infection and even possibly the cause of a stroke in some patients. Some particular types of strokes, for example, hemorrhage into the lobes and some of the deeper structures, are associated with fever as a secondary event.

Aside from these situations, fever in and of itself is associated with worse outcomes in stroke patients. This probably has to do with the fact that higher temperatures lead to increased metabolic activity. The higher the metabolic activity, the more oxygen and glucose the body needs, and, in a stroke, these two substances are exactly what are lacking. Therefore, it is important to treat fever and lower the temperature in all stroke patients, regardless of the source of the fever. Doctors use antipyretics (fever-lowering medicines) and cooling blankets to accomplish this.

Given the reason that fever is bad for stroke, some readers may wonder whether artificially lowering the body temperature even below normal would help. In fact, this has been tried but with disappointing results, and, as of now, creating hypothermia is not recommended for stroke patients.

PAIN AND ANXIETY

Just as in any patient, treating pain and anxiety is important. In stroke patients in particular, it is even more important, because acute pain and/or anxiety is another factor that can raise the blood pressure. In fact, treating the headache of a patient with a hemorrhagic stroke may result in a decreased blood pressure, which may be beneficial to that person. It is also important to address the person's anxiety; having a stroke can be a very scary event. This is especially likely if the patient cannot speak properly. Treating anxiety does not necessarily mean giving medicine; sometimes simply discussing the patient's condition, addressing their concerns, and informing them what is being done is all that is required. If medications were used, it would be important to use very low doses that, ideally, would not affect the individual's mental status so that the effects of the medications would not become confused with the effects of the stroke.

BLOOD SUGAR

Blood sugar, or blood glucose, is another important concept. In diabetic patients, elevated blood sugar is the key chemical finding, but, in patients who undergo various physiological stresses, such as trauma, heart attack, surgery, or stroke, the blood sugar may also become elevated. In these cases, the elevated blood sugar is not a sign of diabetes but of physiological stress.

Over the past decade or so, doctors have learned that stroke patients with high blood sugar levels, in general, have more severe strokes. They have also learned that stroke patients with high blood sugar have worse outcomes and higher fatality rates. This is true even in nondiabetic patients. There is also evidence that stroke patients with higher blood sugar expand the amount of tissue that is involved. This may seem counterintuitive because sugar is one of the things that the brain is being deprived of, but the data are pretty clear.

Less clear are the effects of reducing blood sugar levels in stroke patients and what the target levels should be. There are studies that are currently in progress to try to find the answers to these questions, but, for now, most doctors will give insulin to stroke patients to keep the blood sugar from getting too far out of control.

Before leaving the concept of elevated blood sugar, remember that too low a blood sugar is also bad for the brain, so monitoring the level of blood sugar on both the high and low sides is important in stroke care.

STROKE CENTERS

The concept of a coronary care unit (CCU) for heart attack victims began in the 1960s. Before that, heart attack patients were treated along with everyone else. The notion of a specialized unit in hospitals did not even exist before the 1960s. Putting knowledgeable doctors and nurses in the same space along with specialized equipment was a totally new concept back then that has become the norm today. For stroke care, the notion of "stroke centers" is a relatively new one. Over the past decade, clinicians, politicians, public health planners, and regulators have placed emphasis on the creation of stroke centers, which will continue to improve outcomes for stroke patients in coming years.

There are two types of stroke centers: primary and comprehensive. Just about any hospital with the desire and resources can be a primary stroke center. Primary stroke centers must have a hospital administration that will commit the financial and personnel resources toward caring for stroke patients. They must have an ED open twenty-four hours a day, seven days a week, along with radiology and clinical laboratories that are also ready to support the doctors in the ED at a moment's notice.

Primary stroke centers must also have a designated "stroke team": a group of people who respond to incoming patients. These individuals need not be extra staff who come in particularly for the potential stroke patient but simply the nurses and doctors already working. Using written care plans, or clinical protocols, these clinicians will go through a checklist approach to confirm the diagnosis of stroke and then begin some of the time-sensitive treatments as rapidly as possible. Because these stroke centers are designated by various regulatory agencies, the paramedics and ambulance crews know to bring possible stroke patients to these hospitals.

Another aspect of the concept of a stroke center is the educational part. The clinicians are required to undergo some training, and the hospital is often required to periodically examine their results. All of this is with the goal of constantly improving the overall care. As you can imagine, this type of training and retraining results in improved outcomes in stroke patients, and, in fact, research has borne this out. It is important to emphasize that primary stroke centers are not always located in big, urban hospitals with all of the latest equipment but are often in community hospitals. This is important because the majority of care in the United States is delivered in these smaller hospitals, which are more widespread across the country.

Comprehensive stroke centers are those large urban tertiary care hospitals where nearly every possible stroke treatment is available. For example, a primary stroke center may just have a CT scanner available, but the comprehensive stroke center will have MRI and other advanced imaging technologies. A primary stroke center may be required to have neurosurgical backup available within a couple of hours, but the comprehensive stroke center will have these specialists immediately available. Some interventions, such as those that require a microcatheter to be placed into the brain, would not be available in a primary stroke center but would at the comprehensive one.

It is important to acknowledge that important parts of stroke care occur after the emergency portion of the care, and this is part of why stroke centers lead to improved outcomes. Admission to the hospital, and to a stroke center in particular, has specific goals. For example, simply having a standardized set of orders and actions for stroke patients can help. Patients can be observed for complications of both the original stroke and of the treatments that are given. Complications can sometimes be prevented and other times treated early to minimize their impact.

All stroke patients are at risk for various medical complications, although not every patient has a complication. Standardized orders will focus on prevention of blood clots and infections. They ensure that physical therapy and rehabilitation begin early to maximize the ultimate function of the patient. Because some patients lose the ability to swallow in a coordinated manner, these orders aim to ensure that patients can safely swallow before they are fed to reduce the complication of pneumonia. For all patients, this standardized approach will ensure that ample nutrition is being given. All of these factors lead to improved patient outcomes and will be discussed in greater detail in Chapter 10.

The other component that a stroke center offers is expert neurocritical care. The CCU from the 1960s has evolved. Over time, ICUs began to specialize. Surgical, respiratory, vascular, pediatric, and neonatal ICUs were also started. Over the past decade, specialized units for neurological patients have come into being. Because the term "NICU" was already taken for the neonatal ICU, doctors usually refer to the neurocritical care unit simply as the "neuro-ICU".

What is special about all these units is the dedicated staff and equipment. The nurses become more familiar with what is the normal expected course of, for example, an ischemic stroke patient, so that when a patient deviates off

Table 5.1.
Components of a Primary Stroke Center

Administrative support from the hospital
Designated acute stroke team
Written clinical care protocols
Emergency medical systems (pre-hospital and ambulance personnel)
Emergency department open 24/7
Stroke unit (within the inpatient part of the hospital)
Neurosurgical backup services within 2 hours (or a transfer agreement to a hospital
   with neurosurgeons)
Brain imaging, 24/7 (usually CT scan)
Clinical laboratory services, 24/7
Quality improvement effort
Educational programs (for the community and for clinicians)

the expected course, they will alert the doctor sooner. The nurses also become more experienced at using the specialized equipment. In a subarachnoid hemorrhage patient who has an intracranial bolt to measure the ICP, they are more used to how to calibrate it and how to care for the wound site where it enters the skull.

The physicians, too, become more expert. By concentrating similar patients into one location, they can better focus on their problems. Often anesthesiologists will begin to specialize in the critically ill neurological patients and gain experience so as to better recognize and treat a problem early, when it is easier to treat. Examples include precise blood pressure and ICP monitoring, seizure monitoring with electroencephalogram to detect occult seizures, and better respiratory care to prevent pneumonia and to follow oxygenation at the tissue level. There is now a new journal, *Neurocritical Care*, that is devoted just to this field, and gradually, neurocritical care is becoming a distinct discipline. Simply put, these specialized units provide economy of care and concentration of expertise.

In theory, all of this sounds good, but does it work? Do stroke centers actually improve outcomes? A 2007 study in *Lancet* observed more than 11,500 Italian stroke patients, some of whom were treated in stroke centers and others were not. The patients who were treated in stroke centers (as opposed to conventional hospital care) were less likely to die and less likely to be seriously disabled.

In the next two chapters, we discuss some of the specific treatments for both ischemic and hemorrhagic stroke. Before we do that, Tables 5.1 and 5.2 list the various elements of both types of stroke centers.

Table 5.2.
Components of a Comprehensive Stroke Center

Personnel with expertise in the following areas
  Vascular neurology
  Neuro ICU
  Vascular neurosurgery
  Nursing director for stroke program
  Advanced practice nurse(s)
  Vascular surgery
  Diagnostic radiology and neuroradiology
  Interventional/endovascular physician(s)
  Critical care medicine
  Physical medicine and rehabilitation
  Rehabilitation therapy (physical, occupational, speech therapy)
  Staff stroke nurse(s)
  Respiratory therapist(s)
  Swallowing assessment
Diagnostic techniques
  MRI with diffusion and perfusion imaging
  Vascular imaging with MRA/MRV and CT perfusion
  CT angiography and xenon CT
  Digital cerebral angiography and spectrometry scanning
  Transcranial Doppler and positron emission tomography scanning
  Carotid duplex ultrasound
  Transesophageal echocardiography
Surgical and interventional therapies
  Carotid endarterectomy
  Clipping of intracranial aneurysm
  Stenting/angioplasty of carotid, vertebral, and intracranial vessels
  Placement of ventriculostomy drains (to drain CSF)
  Brain hematoma removal/draining
  Placement of intracranial pressure transducer (to measure ICP)
  Endovascular ablation of aneurysms and AVMs
  Intra-arterial reperfusion therapy
  Endovascular treatment of vasospasm (after subarachnoid hemorrhage)
Infrastructure
  Stroke unit
  ICU stroke clinic
  Operating room staffed 24/7 and air ambulance
  Interventional services coverage 24/7 neuroscience ICU
  Stroke registry
Educational/research programs
  Community education and prevention
  Clinical and laboratory research
  Professional education and fellowship program
  Patient education
  Presentations at national meetings

6

Specific Treatment of Ischemic Stroke

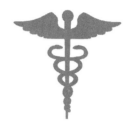

The specific treatment for an ischemic stroke depends in part on how quickly the patient arrives at an ED. A patient who calls 911 within minutes of the onset of their symptoms is rapidly transported to the hospital and undergoes quick evaluation as outlined in Chapter 5. This patient will be treated differently than someone who waits two days to go to the hospital. This is because the most important treatment for acute ischemic stroke is very time sensitive.

FIBRINOLYTIC (THROMBOLYTIC) TREATMENT

This section on thrombolytic therapy is important for many reasons; therefore, we will spend a good deal of time with it. In part, it is important because it represents one of the few Food and Drug Administration (FDA)-approved drugs for ischemic stroke treatment. In addition, it is important because it is a treatment that has been very controversial for nearly fifteen years. Finally, it is an extremely interesting lesson in how science in the real world works.

Remember that ischemic stroke is caused by a blood clot in an artery that feeds a portion of the brain. It is therefore logical that, if doctors were able to successfully break up that clot and restore blood flow, the injured brain might regain its function. To continue that logic, this would theoretically lead to improved patient outcomes. In fact, this is what emergency physicians and heart specialists have been doing for the past twenty years to treat heart attack patients.

However, there are some problems with the theory as it relates to stroke. First of all, the cells of the brain begin to die very quickly, sometimes within minutes, after they are deprived of nutrients. This is different from the heart muscle cells, which are more resilient. The second problem with the theory is that the restoration of blood flow itself can cause problems to the delicate cells that have just undergone a period of oxygen and glucose deprivation. Bleeding and swelling can develop, a problem referred to as "reperfusion injury."

The evolution of this theoretical concept, giving a medication to open the blocked artery in acute ischemic stroke, to an FDA-approved therapy has been nothing short of amazing. It is helpful (not to mention interesting) to understand some of the history of this.

If you accidentally cut yourself, you bleed. Have you ever wondered why the bleeding stops? Were it not for the process of blood coagulation (clotting), you could literally bleed to death from a minor cut. This can happen in some people whose blood coagulation factors don't work properly, such as patients with hemophilia. In normal individuals, the bleeding stops because our coagulation system kicks in and stops the bleeding. But did you ever wonder why the clotting stops? Why doesn't the clotting just keep clotting off every blood vessel in your body?

The answer to these questions is that there is a constant balance between bleeding and clotting. When a blood vessel is injured, a series of chemical events happen that promote clotting. Some of the procoagulant substances that are formed are fibrin and thrombin. When these substances are formed, other chemical reactions naturally start that check the process; these substances are called fibrinolytic or thrombolytic substances because they "lyse" (break up) the clot-promoting chemicals. This remarkable balance is continually occurring, and, when one side or the other is out of balance, we either bleed or we clot too much.

One of the naturally occurring fibrinolytic substances is called tissue plasminogen activator (tPA). There are other fibrinolytic (also called thrombolytic) substances, but for now we will focus just on tPA. tPA can also be manufactured in much larger quantities and used as a medication. You may have heard about this drug, sometimes referred to as a "clot-busting" drug. It is used in patients with heart attacks, large clots in the lungs, and clotted kidney dialysis tubes. Because of the inherent logic of using fibrinolytic medications for ischemic stroke, investigators began experimenting with them as far back as the early 1960s, and since the 1960s, doctors have known that tPA use for ischemic stroke leads to the serious complication of bleeding. The most feared (and the most fatal) site of bleeding is in the brain, in the very area that was involved by the stroke in the first place.

By giving large (pharmacological) doses rather than tiny (physiological) doses of a fibrinolytic agent, Mother Nature's balance can be upset to favor bleeding. Also remember the concept of reperfusion injury. If the clot is successfully dissolved, then a rush of blood will "reperfuse" the area of stroke, sending a high-pressure surge of blood into a place where the brain cells are still not working normally. This also probably contributes to the bleeding.

Suffice it to say that as early as the 1960s, doctors suspected that tPA (or drugs like it) could dissolve the stroke-causing clot but, at the same time, could result in often-fatal bleeding into the brain. They needed to proceed but with great caution. In the late 1980s, stroke neurologists began to plan large-scale trials that would test two different specific fibrinolytic medications: streptokinase and tPA. They began conducting these trials in the early 1990s. Streptokinase was frequently used to treat heart attacks during that era. Three separate studies (Australian Streptokinase Study, Multicenter Acute Stroke Trial–Italy [MAST-I], and Multicenter Acute Stroke Trial–Europe [MAST-E]; see below) asked the question, "would streptokinase lead to improved outcomes in patients with acute ischemic stroke?"

All of these studies had the same basic model. All of the patients were diagnosed by a doctor as having had a stroke. They then had a brain CT scan that showed no hemorrhage and next would be given either the drug being tested or a placebo. Which treatment was given to which patient was done randomly, and neither the doctor nor the patient knew who was given a particular treatment. Thus, these were randomized, double-blinded studies, the best kind in terms of methodological design. The measures of interest were also similar in all the studies. What was the death rate? What was the hemorrhage rate? And how were the neurological outcomes?

For neurological outcomes, there were four different scales that were used. We will learn more about these in Chapter 10. For now, know that three of the scales are measures of how well patients can do various activities of day-to-day life. The fourth scale is the NIHSS (a measure of the neurological physical examination) that we learned about in Chapter 4.

There was much enthusiasm that these trials would show that this new therapy that had such favorable results in heart attack patients would also help stroke patients, but the results of all three of these studies (which were all published between 1995 and 1996) were surprising: all three showed an excess mortality rate in the streptokinase-treated patients. Remarkably, all three of the studies were terminated sooner than planned because the increase in the mortality caused by the fibrinolytic drug was so prominent! Then also published in 1995, the results of a fourth trial were announced (European Cooperative Acute Stroke Study [ECASS]; see below), this one using tPA, and this study also showed lack of benefit of the medication in the original patients.

All four of these major studies showed a dramatic increase in bleeding in the brain from the fibrinolytic medications.

As you might have imagined, the enthusiasm for fibrinolytic treatment of stroke dampened. Just as important, there were rifts that were forming within as well as between different groups of investigators. One of the landmark streptokinase papers, MAST-I, was published in *Lancet*, a major international medical journal. Two of the investigators went to the extraordinary measure of removing their support for the publication and writing a separate "dissenting" editorial in the same issue of the journal. We won't go into the details here because they have to do with the methodological design of the study, but suffice it to say that this degree of disagreement between doctors in the same investigative group is nearly unprecedented.

During the same years that these four trials were being accomplished in Europe, U.S. investigators were also busy with a National Institutes of Health (NIH)-sponsored trial of tPA for stroke. This study (which was actually two closely related but separate studies) was done by the National Institute of Neurological Disorders and Stroke (NINDS). The first part was to treat patients with stroke and see how much improvement there was at twenty-four hours after therapy. Basically, the investigators would measure the NIHSS before and then twenty-four hours after tPA treatment. In Part Two of the study, investigators would measure different measures of neurological outcomes at three months, as well as any bleeding into the brain and mortality.

In December 1995, the NINDS study, as it was called, was published in the prestigious *New England Journal of Medicine*. Part One of the study was a "negative" study; that is to say, it did not show any positive effect of tPA on the NIHSS at twenty-four hours after giving the drug. Put another way, the neurological examination at twenty-four hours had not substantially changed any more or less in treated, than in untreated, patients.

However, Part Two of the NINDS trial was "positive." It showed an improvement in the conditions of the patients as measured by the various metrics. In fact, it showed a fairly robust improvement: approximately 12 percent absolute improvement. This means that, for every one hundred patients treated with tPA, about twelve additional patients would be normal or near normal compared with the placebo group. This may not sound like a large number, but in the world of medical research, it is quite significant.

Some were elated to finally have a positive thrombolytic trial in stroke, but others were extremely cautious. After all, the three streptokinase trials had all been prematurely terminated because of excess mortality in drug-treated patients, and the other trial using tPA also failed to show benefit. Add to that the fact that Part One of NINDS was a negative trial that caused many physicians (neurologists, emergency physicians, and others) to view the NINDS Part Two with a great deal of suspicion.

It is important to highlight the inequalities of these early trials because some used different medications, different doses, and different time windows and allowed other anti-clotting drugs to be given at the same time. Table 6.1 illustrates these differences.

A general principle of the scientific method is the reproducibility of one scientist's work by another. This means that, if one scientist performs an experiment, he should be able to describe his methods in sufficient detail such that another scientist, at another place in another laboratory, should be able to duplicate those same methods and that both experiments would show the same result. One of the corollaries of this point is that the experimental design has everything controlled except for a single variable that is being tested.

In the ideal world, if the experiment were about thrombolytics in ischemic stroke, then the drug would be the same one at the same dose that was given in the same time window from onset of symptoms. Other variables (such as aspirin or other drugs that could affect the results) would be controlled to be the same. The patients would be similar in age and various risk factors such as diabetes and hypertension. The radiologists interpreting the CT scans would all be of equal skill level and have the same threshold for reading a hemorrhage or not. All these principles would be applied to the countless variables that exist in such a complex experiment. However, as you can see from Table 6.1, there were significant differences in the first five major thrombolytic studies.

Table 6.1.
Comparison of the Early Trials of Thrombolytic Drugs for Stroke

Trial	Thrombolytic used	Dose	Time window	Other drugs allowed
ASK	Streptokinase	1.5 mU	4 hours	No
MAST-I	Streptokinase	1.5 mU	6 hours	Yes (aspirin)
MAST-E	Streptokinase	1.5 mU	6 hours	No
ECASS	tPA	1.1 mg/kg	3 hours	No
NINDS	tPA	0.9 mg/kg	3 hours	No

Because of the principle of science that states that results must be reproducible, many doctors were unconvinced by the single positive study (NINDS). Others, in comparison, were ready to declare tPA as a therapy that should be used for ischemic stroke. As you can imagine, a great controversy arose.

In June 1996, just six months after the NINDS results were published, the FDA licensed tPA for use in acute ischemic stroke. Some stroke doctors were glad to finally have an FDA-approved treatment for a disease that formerly had none. However, others were appalled. How could this national regulatory agency license a drug about which there was so much controversy and so much scientific doubt? Not only was the evidence based solely on one study that had not been reproduced by other investigators, but there was plenty of contrary data from the other four early trials!

In addition, there were issues with the methods in the NINDS trials that some complained about. There was the fact that the trial, although sponsored by the NIH, was manufacturer supported (and the drug company had undue influence). There were also concerns about the tenfold increase in intracerebral hemorrhage (ICH) in the patients treated with tPA.

Some argued that there was the possibility that the therapeutic effect of tPA was simply attributable to chance. This gets back to the reason of why trials must be duplicated, to make sure that the play of chance has been excluded. Consider the following experiment. If you flip a coin ten times, it is certainly possible that you will get ten consecutive heads, because for each individual flip, there is a 50:50 chance that is independent of the other nine times that you flip the coin. If you happened, by sheer chance, to throw ten consecutive heads tosses, you could come up with the incorrect conclusion that there is a 100 percent chance that when you toss a coin, it will land in the heads position.

However, if you were to replicate this experiment, or have a friend do it, you would quickly find that the conclusion simply is not true: that if you continued to flip the coin (or another coin), some tails would come up, and, if you flipped it 1,000 times, the percentage of heads would be very close to 50 percent.

There was a great deal of "hype" with tPA use. Even the AHA made the incorrect statement that tPA "saves lives," when in fact, although the NINDS trial showed that tPA led to improved outcomes, there was no statistically significant evidence of reduced mortality. When this point was brought out, the AHA backed off on this erroneous claim. In addition, in 2000, the AHA elevated its support of tPA for ischemic stroke by labeling it "standard of care" or "level 1" evidence, all of this once again based on a single trial. Importantly, it was discovered that the manufacturer of tPA, Genentech, had donated more than $11 million to the AHA over the preceding ten years. Many doctors thought that this financial relationship was improper, especially because it had not been fully disclosed by the AHA.

Our purpose here is not to debate the ethics of this relationship, but you can see the backdrop to the controversy about tPA use for stroke.

Over the decade that followed the NINDS study, other studies were published showing that tPA use in routine community practice (not by stroke specialists in the large studies) had worse outcomes than that reported in the trials done at larger academic settings. It is one thing to be able to get certain results in the environment of a controlled clinical trial with experts watching every phase of care. It is quite another to translate this into routine practice in which the same treatment is often far more difficult to implement. As a result, by 2000 or so, there were various organizations that held very different views about tPA use in stroke.

The AHA and the American Academy of Neurologists developed policy statements supporting its routine use. However, the American College of Emergency Physicians, the Society for Academic Emergency Physicians, and the American Association of Emergency Physicians had all issued statements that tPA was not standard care in all practice settings. For all of these reasons, tPA was used very infrequently in the United States.

The situation in other countries was similar. In Canada, tPA was not licensed until 1999 and in Europe not until 2002. In both of these countries, a condition of licensure by the regulatory organization was that a registry of cases be maintained to ensure that the safety and effectiveness in routine use could match the performance seen in large studies. These registries from Canada and Europe have just been published in the past few years. Both showed results in routine practice that did match those from the big studies.

As of 2007, most neurologists and many emergency physicians believe that tPA is useful in acute ischemic stroke, but some controversy still exists. With all that said, the use of tPA is, in the opinion of the author, a safe and effective treatment for patients who can be treated in less than three hours from onset of symptoms and in a setting that pays great care to the details of the various diagnostic and therapeutic steps. This is not an easy thing to do, however, because the patient must recognize that there is a problem, activate 911, get to the hospital, have the hospital personnel recognize that the patient may be having a stroke, get the CT scan to exclude a hemorrhage (and have it interpreted), ensure that there are no conditions that would make tPA use unsafe (such as blood thinning medications, a brain tumor, or many other factors), and then finally give the tPA. This is a lot to accomplish in a short period of time, but it is certainly doable if all goes right.

FIBRINOLYTIC TREATMENT BEYOND THREE HOURS FROM ONSET OF SYMPTOMS

Analysis of some of the evidence from these large trials suggests a favorable effect beyond three hours from onset of symptoms. As of 2007, there are ongoing trials that are testing the possibility that tPA given between three and four and a half hours is still effective, but, as of the current time, the tPA is only licensed to be given in the first three hours. Hopefully, we will know in a few years when all the data has been collected and analyzed whether tPA is useful beyond three hours.

The one exception is that sometimes the drug can be given intra-arterially rather than intravenously (all of the previous information in this chapter refers to intravenous use). Some physicians have been using tPA given through an artery.

In this procedure, a specialist will take the patient to a catheterization lab as one would for a heart attack patient. Again, just like for a heart attack patient, a tiny flexible catheter is inserted into the femoral artery in the groin and then, under x-ray guidance, is fed up the body, through the main artery (aorta), and into the carotid or vertebral arteries that feed the brain. A small amount of dye is then injected into the artery to find the site of the blockage, and then the tPA (in smaller dosages) is injected directly at the site of the blockage. Although this is not standard therapy, some physicians are using it because it can be given after the narrow three-hour window. We will discuss intra-arterial use of tPA in Chapter 11 because, at the present time, it is not an FDA-approved and routine therapy.

While we are on the subject of "brain catheterization," there are some other strategies that the specialist can try in the catheterization lab (see Figure 6.1). Using the same equipment and techniques described above, the doctor can deploy tiny devices that are like mini-corkscrews that can literally pull the clot out. The corkscrew is "screwed" into the clot and then the clot is withdrawn through the catheter. This is known as an "endovascular" technique, doing a procedure from within the blood vessel. We will talk much more about this in Chapter 7 when we discuss the treatment of brain aneurysms. It is certainly possible that, over time, new endovascular techniques will be developed and used. We will discuss this more in Chapter 11.

ANTICOAGULATION DRUG THERAPY

We have discussed fibrinolytic drugs, but there are also anticoagulant medications. The primary drug in this class is called heparin. Heparin differs from the thrombolytic drugs. It does not dissolve the clot; it simply stops new clots from forming. Because such a large percentage of ischemic strokes are caused by clots, it is logical that heparin would be useful to treat them.

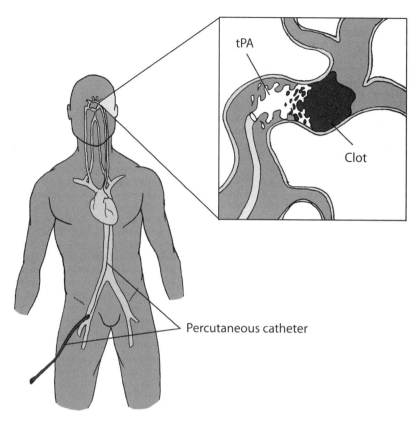

Percutaneous catheter

Figure 6.1. Illustration of how a "brain catheterization" works. The operator inserts a catheter into the femoral artery in the groin and threads it up into the artery necessary (usually the carotid but sometimes the vertebral). When the catheter is in the correct location, the doctor will squirt some dye that shows up on the x-ray to know both the location and the status of the artery (e.g., whether it is blocked, whether there is a dissection, etc.). In the inset, the doctor is administering intra-arterial tPA to dissolve a clot. This same general procedure is used for all endovascular treatments such as the corkscrew clot extractor described above.

There have been many trials that have examined this indication for heparin and its cousin, low-molecular-weight heparin. None of these trials have shown that any of the heparin-type drugs are useful in acute ischemic stroke. Heparin is useful to prevent strokes, especially in patients with atrial fibrillation. We will discuss this indication for heparin at greater length in the chapters on stroke prevention and treatment of TIA.

There are other anticoagulation drugs. There are oral ones such as Coumadin, and there are experimental drugs such as those derived from bat saliva and pit viper venom. At the present time, these have no place in the routine treatment of acute stroke, but again, these drugs will come up in subsequent chapters.

ANTI-PLATELET DRUG THERAPY

The situation with anti-platelet drugs is a bit complicated. Remember that, in the streptokinase trials, the co-use of aspirin, which is the most commonly used anti-platelet drug, could result in worse outcomes. Therefore, the current standard is that, if a patient is eligible to be treated with a thrombolytic drug, aspirin (or other anti-platelet drugs) is not given.

However, what about the situation for patients who are not eligible for tPA, a far larger group of patients? Two very large trials with thousands of patients have shown that simple aspirin given shortly after the start of stroke symptoms results in improved outcomes. This is an important point. Because aspirin is so inexpensive and because it can be used in the vast majority of patients, the public health impact of aspirin in ischemic stroke is far greater than the impact of tPA. In these two large trials, tens of thousands of patients were randomized to receive either aspirin or placebo after ischemic strokes.

Both of these studies found the same result; approximately ten patients per 1,000 treated with aspirin will avoid death or severe strokes. Interventions that might produce smaller effects, but that can be applied to large numbers of individuals because of simplicity and low cost, have a very large effect on a population.

NEUROPROTECTIVE AGENTS

The concept of a neuroprotective drug is a medicine that can be given after the onset of a stroke that protects individual brain cells from dying after the injury from the stroke. Literally hundreds of neuroprotective agents have been tested on laboratory animals, and many of these have gone on to be tested in clinical trials on humans. Thus far, none of these neuroprotective drugs have been found to be effective. We will discuss the concept of new therapies a bit more in Chapter 11, but in this chapter, we will discuss one neuroprotectant drug because the lessons learned from it help to better understand the controversy about tPA.

The most recent drug to undergo a full-fledged clinical trial was an agent called NXY-059. This is a typical name of a drug that is still experimental; only later, when a drug is brought to the market, is it given a catchier, "trade" name. NXY-059 was developed by the AstraZeneca pharmaceutical company and seemed to work well in animal experiments. Then it was tested in a large human trial, again with favorable results. These results were greeted with a great deal of anticipation. AstraZeneca began to do marketing research, and there was much hype amongst doctors who were ready for another way to suc-cessfully treat ischemic stroke. Some hoped that neuroprotectants might increase the time window during which thrombolytic drugs were useful. The company even gave the fledgling drug a name, Cerovive.

After the animal and initial human trials were published, a phase 3 trial was required. A phase 3 trial is one that is FDA required that would prove the effectiveness of Cerovive. Phase 1 studies are the first investigations that come early in the process of developing a new drug. These initial studies try to determine the right dose and make sure it can be absorbed. They also test how long it remains in the body and whether it is eliminated by the liver or by the kidneys. Phase 2 trials are safety trials. These studies are larger studies that involve a larger number of patients and are done with an eye for defining the safety profile of the experimental agent. Phase 3 trials are even larger, often double-blinded randomized trials that are meant to definitively test how well a drug actually works. Phase 4 trials are generally done after a drug is approved to test the safety and efficacy of the drug in routine practice. The FDA often mandates these phase 4 studies. The large studies, or registries of tPA done in Canada and Europe mentioned above, are examples of phase 4 studies.

With respect to Cerovive (NXY-059) the results surprised everyone. After promising results in earlier trials, the phase 3 trial was negative! That is to say, it showed that the drug did not significantly improve outcomes. This is a great example of why there was appropriate reluctance when the NINDS trial showed a favorable result in the face of all the other articles that were nega-tive. As well, it again illustrates the importance of the principle of science that results must be reproducible for them to be believable and useful.

This escapade also shows, at least in part, why pharmaceutical drugs cost so much money. After the many millions of dollars spent to develop NXY-059, in the end, AstraZeneca had to drop it. Although most drugs do not get this far into the pipeline before the investigators realize they do not work, some do. Built into the cost of drugs that do ultimately work is the research and develop-ment for drugs that show initial promise but then are found to be worthless.

LIPIDS

Over time, doctors have become much more aggressive about treating high blood lipid levels (cholesterol and triglycerides) in stroke patients. This falls more logically into the realm of stroke prevention (because the treatment has been found to reduce recurrent stroke, not as treatment of the stroke per se). There-fore, we will cover this study and this topic in the chapter on stroke prevention.

7

Treatment of Hemorrhagic Stroke

As we learned in previous chapters, there are many causes for hemorrhagic stroke, and, not surprisingly, the treatments vary depending on the cause. In this chapter, we will discuss the treatments based on the causes. To refresh our memory, we will repeat the list of causes here (see Table 7.1). This list differs slightly from the chart in Chapter 2 in that the causes are listed more based on order of importance. As well, there are two kinds of intracranial bleeding (subdural and epidural hematomas) that are not really strokes in the traditional sense of the word but can present like one and so will be included here for completeness. However, before we go through this diagnosis-related list, there are some general principles of intracranial bleeding and its treatment that we will discuss first.

GENERAL ISSUES

As a general rule, the treatment of hemorrhagic stroke has been much more surgical than medical. It makes sense that, if there is extra blood that is outside of blood vessels and that is compressing normal brain tissue within the confines of a tight box (the skull), then draining out the blood would be a helpful thing to do. However, with one exception that we will discuss in Chapter 11, ischemic stroke is not a pathologic process that surgery can help.

Table 7.1.
Causes of Hemorrhagic Stroke

Amyloid angiopathy
Hypertensive bleed
Intracranial aneurysm
Coagulopathy-associated bleeding
AVM (and other vascular abnormalities)
Venous sinus thrombosis
Arterial dissection
Vasculitis
Subdural hemorrhage
Epidural hemorrhage

Brain surgery is high tech to be sure, but archeological evidence from Europe, Egypt, and Central America shows that successful brain surgery was being done thousands of years before the birth of Christ. Skulls have been found with very precise holes and with subsequent growth of bone that followed the time that the hole was made, indicating that these "patients" survived the procedure, at least for weeks to months. It is not clear what the purpose was of these procedures, and some archeologists believe that some were done for religious or spiritual reasons. However, archeological evidence exists that suggests that some of these operations were attempted for medical reasons.

Although the techniques, the anesthesia, and the treatment of pain and infection have made obvious and substantial gains over those of ancient times, the most basic principles are the same: drain the blood (or tumor or infection) that is pressing on properly functioning brain tissue so that the good tissue is preserved. Over the past century, with the development of modern neurosurgical techniques, neurosurgeons have frequently operated on patients with brain bleeds.

Figure 7.1 shows a typical intracranial hemorrhage. In the figure, the blood exerts pressure on nearby tissue. The more blood, the greater the pressure. The greater the pressure, the more distortion there is of normal brain structures. The skull is noncompressible. In Chapter 5, we touched briefly on the concept of ICP. Remember that the contents of the skull (brain, venous and arterial blood, and CSF) exert a certain amount of expected pressure. As this pressure is exceeded, there are a limited number of ways in which the average individual's brain will compensate. Some of the venous blood will get "pushed" out, and, to some extent, the CSF can also be pushed into the subarachnoid space in the back.

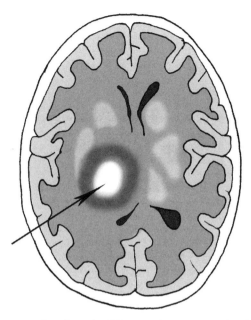

Figure 7.1. A representative slice of a CT scan of a patient with a hypertensive intracranial hemorrhage (arrow). Note that there is pressure on the structures that are adjacent to the bleed and that there is a thin rim of (darker gray) swelling around the bleeding.

It is easy to see, given the volume of blood shown in Figure 7.1, that those compensatory mechanisms will only go so far. Normal brain tissue will be pushed against the skull and the firm portion of the meninges (the dura). This pressure can either alter function or, if severe enough, kill the affected portion of brain tissue. Also, the pressure caused by the blood can twist blood vessels that are still intact, which can add an ischemic insult to the hemorrhagic injury. Last, some portions of the brain, especially the brainstem, can also be twisted and deformed, resulting in diminished function. Because parts of the brainstem are instrumental in the function of the heartbeat, in breathing, and even in maintaining consciousness, this latter problem can be fatal.

When a portion of the brain is pushed and distorted by pressure from within the skull, this abnormal process is called "herniation." Herniation is one cause of death after a stroke, more commonly in a hemorrhagic stroke.

So there are three kinds of therapy that, to some extent, are general to all kinds of hemorrhagic stroke: surgery (to reduce the pressure), procoagulant medicines (to stop the bleeding), and interventions to reduce ICP (to decrease the likelihood of herniation or to treat elevated ICP if it already exists).

SURGERY

For decades (or for millennia if you count the Egyptians), surgeons have done surgery to drain the blood from the brain. This is important for the obvious reason of diminishing the volume of blood and thereby reducing the pressure but also to try to decrease the bleeding that occurs after the initial hemorrhage. By doing sequential CT scans on hemorrhagic stroke patients over the first forty-eight hours, doctors have learned that almost 40 percent of these patients have an increase in the size of the bleed (by more than one-third) over the first three hours. In fact, often the increased bleeding occurred in the first hour after diagnosis. Not surprisingly, patients whose bleeding increased had higher death rates, and those who survived had worse outcomes. So the surgeon can not only remove the blood that has already bled but cauterize or in some manner treat the oozing blood vessel to prevent future bleeding.

The logic in this approach is undeniable, and, in some cases, it clearly works. In part, because of the inherent logic, for a long time, no one ever did an actual scientific study to see whether surgery helped over simple management with medicines and all the other general measures that we discussed in Chapter 5. Some small studies had been done, but they were not large enough to draw meaningful conclusions. In 1995, neurosurgeons from 107 institutions in a number of countries began to study this issue. They ultimately recruited more than 1,000 patients with ICH to be randomized to have surgery or to not have surgery. So the Surgical Treatment for Intracranial Hemorrhage (STICH) was a randomized trial, but not of a drug like tPA but a surgical procedure. In and of itself, organizing and completing this large study that involved so many individuals was a huge accomplishment.

Overall, the STICH study that found that the long-held notion that surgery was useful for most intracranial bleeding has been seriously questioned. Operated patients were no better off than those treated medically (that is, without surgery). Like most big studies, there were some weaknesses in STICH, which were serious ones. Some of the "early" surgery patients did not have their operation for one to three days after their stroke, and some of them never even had surgery. As well, some of the patients randomized to nonsurgical treatment ended up having surgery.

One finding was that patients who started out comatose did better with medical rather than surgical treatment. Patients whose bleeding was close to the surface of the brain did better than patients whose bleeding was deeper. It is worth noting that patients with cerebellar hemorrhages were excluded from the study because most neurosurgeons believe that all but the smallest of these bleeds need to be operated on, and it would not have been ethical to include these patients in the STICH study.

Although the STICH study answered some questions, it left many unanswered, and neurosurgeons still must decide on a case-by-case basis which patients may benefit from early operation and which patients are best treated medically.

PROCOAGULANT MEDICATIONS

If bleeding is the underlying problem, then administering a medication that will make blood less thin, or more likely to clot, also has some intrinsic logic to treat patients with ICH. A procoagulant drug is one that makes blood clot more easily.

There are two situations in which this can be used. The first is patients who start off with a problem in blood coagulation. Sometimes, this occurs with a disease, such as hemophilia or liver disease from excess alcohol intake or hepatitis. The other, which is far more common, is in patients who take anticoagulant medications to treat some underlying condition. One of the most common, as we have seen earlier, is atrial fibrillation. We discussed this in the chapter on risk factors and will discuss it again in the chapter on prevention. Suffice it to say that the treatment for one condition (atrial fibrillation, which predisposes one to ischemic stroke) can be a risk factor for another type of stroke (hemorrhagic).

The other situation in which a procoagulant drug could be used is any hemorrhagic stroke at all, even if the patient is not taking an anticoagulant (or has an intrinsic disease affecting his coagulation system). This is a far more interesting situation because this could be given to all patients with hemorrhagic stroke if it worked.

This was tested recently with a drug called Factor 7 (which is a natural blood-clotting factor that we all have). This drug was tested in an early trial by giving it to patients who were not on anticoagulant medications. In a phase 2 trial, the drug appeared to work. Phase 1 trials test the drug for safety in closely monitored human volunteers. A phase 2 trial is a randomized trial to test the drug's effectiveness in the condition or illness being treated. Phase 3 trials are larger, better designed randomized trials to best answer the clinical question that is being asked.

For Factor 7 in intracranial hemorrhage, there were meaningful improvements not only in the amount of blood found by CT scans but also some clinical improvements in the outcome of patients. This phase 2 trial was sufficiently important that is was published in the prestigious *New England Journal of Medicine*. Because of the excellent results and the high-profile publication, there was great expectation for the phase 3 study.

However, once again, as we saw with the NXY-059 neuroprotectant drug, the phase 3 trial was unable to reproduce the results of the previous study, and the manufacturer backed off on its development. However, the fact that Factor 7 did not work does not mean that other procoagulant medicines will not work in the future.

INTERVENTIONS TO REDUCE ICP

The third generic way to treat various types of hemorrhagic stroke has to do with several interventions designed to reduce ICP. Some of these interventions are so simple that the very word intervention seems a bit over the top. For example, keeping the head of the bed elevated by thirty degrees can improve the venous drainage from the brain, thereby keeping pressure down. Another is making sure that the head and neck are straight and that there is no constrictive clothing at the neck. Both of these can also help venous blood flow out of the brain and reduce ICP. Other simple measures include adequately treating pain and anxiety, as mentioned previously.

Some of the measures are more high tech. One of them is to administer a medication called mannitol. Mannitol is a large sugar molecule that helps to reduce ICP by reducing brain swelling. By osmotic pressure, the large sugar molecule pulls out excess brain water. This can only work temporarily.

Another method is called hyperventilation. For this to be successful, doctors must sedate the patient and place a breathing tube into the trachea. Then, the patient is put on an artificial breathing machine called a ventilator. Next, the machine will breathe at a faster than physiologic rate and push more air in during each breath. Hyperventilation will cause the arteries in the brain to constrict. As we learned before, if one component of intracranial contents (in this case, the arterial blood) decreases, the ICP goes down. This is a two-edged sword, however, because if the constriction of arteries is too much or goes on for too long, it can lead to brain ischemia.

Both hyperventilation and mannitol can work very well, but because of dangers with both and because both are temporary, they must be used very strategically. Of the other potential treatments (CSF drainage with a catheter, medication-induced coma, and/or paralysis), none has been convincingly shown to be effective.

AMYLOID ANGIOPATHY

This type of hemorrhagic stroke refers to the abnormal blood vessels that form most commonly in elderly patients. The older a person is, the more likely he or she is to have these changes in their blood vessels. Although it does not mean that all of them will have bleeding, 12 percent of people over age eighty will show these changes, and, as the population ages, this kind of stroke is expected to become far more common. The good news from the STICH trial is that these are just the kind of patients who may benefit from early surgery because the location of bleeding from amyloid angiopathy-related stroke tends to be lobar and in the periphery of the brain. The bad news is that there is currently no specific therapy for the underlying vascular problem, so there is no one medication or intervention to treat those hemorrhagic strokes caused by amyloid angiopathy.

HYPERTENSIVE BLEED

The good news here is that hypertensive bleeds are far less common now than they were twenty years ago. This is attributable to far better treatment of high blood pressure in the general community. There are many reasons for this, and we will discuss some of them in Chapter 9 on prevention. Part of the reason that it is fortunate is that hypertensive bleeds tend to occur in the deeper structures of the brain. As we learned with the STICH study, these deeper bleeds are in general less susceptible to surgical treatment and often lead to severe neurological impairment.

Part of the specific treatment that relates to treating hypertensive hemorrhagic stroke relates back to some basic brain physiology that we learned at the beginning of the book: the principle of CPP. Most patients with hypertensive bleeds have had their high blood pressure for many years, if not decades. Their cerebral circulation is used to these high perfusion pressures, and so any attempt to reduce these patients' blood pressures too low can be disastrous. Their pressure can drop too low, and, instead of making the situation better, the brain does not get enough flow and parts of the brain become ischemic, again, adding (an ischemic) insult to (hemorrhagic) injury.

One part of the brain that hypertensive strokes have a predilection for is the cerebellum. As we learned, the cerebellum is that back portion of the brain that relates to balance and agility. It is also the part of the brain that is in the tightest area, the posterior fossa. Therefore, when patients have cerebellar hemorrhage from hypertension, this is one of the most time-sensitive neurosurgical emergencies that there is. Remember that, in the STICH trial, which showed generally unfavorable results for surgical drainage of ICH, cerebellar hemorrhage patients were excluded from even being entered into the trial.

COAGULOPATHY-ASSOCIATED BLEED

Increasing numbers of patients are being treated with anticoagulant medications. The most common are warfarin (or Coumadin) and anti-platelet drugs (such as aspirin and clopidogrel). There is a price to pay for any medicine that anticoagulates the blood, and that price is bleeding. Nowhere in the body is that price higher than bleeding into the brain. This type of ICH is clearly increasing over time and, even now, represents an important cause of hemorrhagic stroke. There is good reason to believe that patients with this kind of bleeding are really just patients who have another reason to bleed (such as hypertension-related or amyloid angiopathy-related bleeds) that is made worse by the anticoagulation.

The specific treatment for this kind of bleeding, in part, depends on what the underlying anticoagulant is. For example, a patient bleeding from aspirin is not going to respond to the same treatment for patients on warfarin. For the most part, in discussing this topic, we are talking about ICH associated with warfarin. The major therapeutic strategy here is to reverse the clotting problem as soon as possible so that the underlying cause of the bleeding will stop. These patients are very difficult to operate on because, even if the surgeon can get to the bleeding area, all the cut surfaces continue to bleed because of the lack of clotting that exists.

Because warfarin interferes with vitamin K-dependent clotting factors, the two therapeutic strategies are to either give back vitamin K or to give back the clotting factors that have been depleted. Vitamin K can be given as a simple intravenous dose, but it takes many hours for the vitamin K to be translated into higher levels of clotting factors because they have to be manufactured in the liver. So this treatment is easy to do but takes time to have its effect and can lead to rare but serious allergic reactions.

Giving back the clotting factors can be done in various ways. The traditional method is to give fresh frozen plasma. This plasma, which is a blood product, contains all the depleted clotting factors, and thus their levels begin to increase as soon as the plasma is given (also administered intravenously). The downside here is that it takes time to get it from the blood bank, it requires large volumes of fluid to be given (which could harm some elderly patients with coexistent heart problems), and there are the usual side effects of any blood-product transfusion (infections and allergic reactions). The other ways of giving back the clotting factors (prothrombin concentrates and other clotting factor concentrates) are very quick and fairly well tolerated but extraordinarily expensive to give. Therefore, they have not yet become standard medical practice.

INTRACRANIAL ANEURYSM

The treatment of intracranial aneurysms has undergone a true revolution in the past two decades. Aneurysms are tiny bubbles or outpouchings on arteries. Figure 7.2 shows an aneurysm before and after clipping. When they occur in the brain, they are usually on large- and mid-sized arteries that lie within the subarachnoid space. The walls of these aneurysms become weaker as they expand, just like the wall of a balloon gets increasingly stretched as more air is blown into it. At some point for both balloons and aneurysms, as the pressure on the inside rises above the ability of the wall (of the balloon or aneurysm to contain it), they rupture.

When an aneurysm ruptures, a tiny amount of blood escapes into the sub-arachnoid space, which is why this is called a subarachnoid hemorrhage. If the bleeding does not stop within seconds, the patient dies, and, in fact, about 10–15 percent of subarachnoid hemorrhage patients do die suddenly. On the other end of the spectrum, in the majority of patients who suffer from this type of hemorrhage, a very small amount of blood leaks and the aneurysm almost instantly clots off. These patients will just have an acute, severe headache, albeit one unlike any headache they have ever had before.

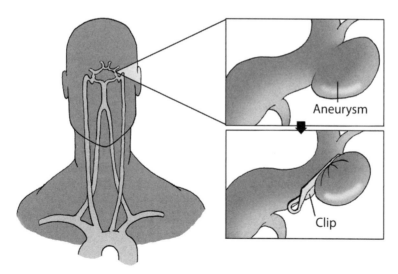

Figure 7.2. A magnified view of an aneurysm bulging off the parent artery (top panel). The bottom panel shows what the surgical clips look like when they are applied to the base of the aneurysm. For patients who have already had a bleed, the clip effectively isolates the aneurysm so that it cannot rerupture and cause a catastrophic second hemorrhage. For patients whose aneurysms are discovered before they rupture, the clip will prevent a subarachnoid hemorrhage.

For most of the past century, the treatment of subarachnoid hemorrhage (the condition that occurs when an aneurysm ruptures), has been surgical. There were variations on the theme (different equipment and different strategies as to where to place the equipment), but basically, the treatment was surgical. The neurosurgeon would do one of several operations. Sometimes, he would place a clip over the carotid artery to reduce the pressure in the artery feeding the aneurysm, thereby hoping to reduce the likelihood of rupture. Other times, he would literally wrap the aneurysm with a material that would decrease the likelihood of rupture.

Over time, especially with the advent of the operating microscope, better methods of isolating the aneurysm from the rest of the cerebrovascular circulation were developed. The operating microscope is a regular microscope that has sterile coverings and that is mobile enough to be swung into the surgical field. Using this microscope, the neurosurgeon can see in exquisite detail all the relevant anatomy: the aneurysm, the arteries that supply it with blood as well as any arteries that drain from the aneurysm, any adjacent structures such as cranial nerves, and other important structures. With the microscope, surgeons can do the operation better and more safely.

With this advancement and with improved methods of anesthesia, neurosurgeons can now apply a surgical clip to most brain aneurysms. Figure 7.2 shows a schematic of how the spring-loaded clip isolates the aneurysm from the rest of the brain circulation. The metal clip is left in place, and this treatment is very durable and has a low failure rate. Surgical clipping, which is still used often, was the standard therapy for aneurysms until the advent of placing endovascular coils into the aneurysm, a revolutionary procedure first used in 1991.

Endovascular (meaning within the blood vessel) embolization, or coiling, uses the natural access to the brain through the bloodstream via arteries to diagnose and treat brain aneurysms. The goal of the treatment is to safely seal off the aneurysm and stop further blood from entering into the aneurysm and increasing the risk of rupture or possibly rebleeding. Figure 7.3 shows a coil that is inside an aneurysm.

The history of this creative procedure is interesting and shows how a single individual can sometimes exert a large influence on medical care. Dr. Guido Guglielmi, an Italian physician, had an interest in electronics and started studying neurology and neurosurgery in Rome. He began studying how the blood in an aneurysm might clot with the application of an electric charge. Then, in 1974, by extraordinary coincidence, his father suffered from a subarachnoid hemorrhage. Over the ensuing fifteen years, Dr. Guglielmi performed numerous experiments until he, along with several colleagues including Dr.

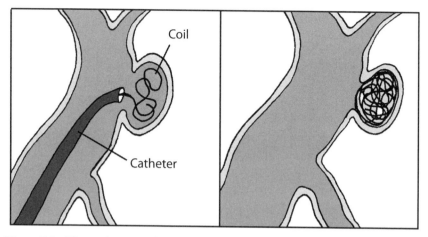

Figure 7.3. The application of a coil into the aneurysm. This newer therapy is being used increasingly to treat both ruptured and nonruptured aneurysms. Using the same endovascular technology for a brain catheterization, the catheter is positioned at the opening of the aneurysm and tiny platinum coils are tightly packed inside. The coils induce thrombosis (clotting) of the blood inside. This clot effectively seals off the aneurysm from the rest of the circulation, thus protecting it from rupture.

Fernando Viñuela at University of California, Los Angeles Medical Center, performed the first application of this new technology in a human being on March 6, 1990. This first patient treated had an abnormal tract, or fistula, in one of the venous sinuses in the brain, and the procedure was a success. The first aneurysm patient was treated in January 1991.

In 1995, the FDA approved the commercial sale of the coil, then called the Guglielmi detachable coil. One interesting footnote to this story pertains to the "detachable" part of the name. The way that the coil was separated from the wire that navigated it to the aneurysm was by the application of a small electrical charge. Dr. Guglielmi first witnessed that phenomenon while doing some related experiments some ten years earlier. At the time, he did not recognize its importance, which would be critical in how the coil is actually deployed into the aneurysm. The work of these men and of course many other colleagues who worked with them on the team would radically change the way aneurysms are "routinely" treated.

At first, these coiling procedures were limited. For one, there were very few individuals who were trained to perform the procedure. Second, because it was so new and because it was quite different from the time-honored surgical approach, doctors were naturally hesitant to begin doing the procedure. Third, in the first few years, the procedure was mostly limited to particular types of aneurysms (such as those with a narrow neck that would help to keep the coils in place; see Figure 7.4) or in patients whose aneurysms were not easily treated surgically because of their location.

Over time, however, more doctors learned how to do this procedure, some of them neuroradiologists, neurosurgeons, and, increasingly, even neurologists with special training. The technology to place the coils has expanded enormously so that aneurysms that previously would have been untreatable with a coil now are. Other devices, such as balloons and stents, can effectively change the vessel anatomy so that coils can be deployed (see Figure 7.4). As well, new materials such as rapidly setting glue-like substances are being used. As the technology and the ability to use it increased, the stage was set for a scientific study of the technique.

As with ICH, there had been some relatively small studies, often reporting on the experience from one hospital done by a single individual. In 2005, the International Study of Aneurysm Treatment was published in the well-respected *Lancet* journal. This study measured outcomes in patients with

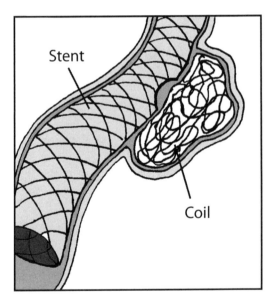

Figure 7.4. An aneurysm that has a very wide neck. Normally, such an aneurysm could not be coiled because the coils would fall back into the parent vessel. In this figure, a stent has first been deployed in the artery. This stent has a small hole through which the coils can be passed. The stent thus converts an aneurysm that could not be coiled into one that can be. This is an example of very sophisticated endovascular technology that was not available just a few years ago.

intracranial aneurysms who were randomized to receive either classical surgical clipping vs. endovascular coiling of intracranial aneurysms. Again, as with all large studies (this one enrolled more than 2,000 patients from dozens of hospitals mostly in Europe), there were some flaws to it, but the bottom line was that patients treated endovascularly had significantly better outcomes than those treated surgically, at least at their one-year follow-up.

It is important to note that, to be included in the study, physicians needed to agree that the aneurysm could be treated by either method, so many patients were excluded because of the location or configuration of their aneurysms. Longer-term follow-up has shown some problems in terms of the durability of the endovascular technique. Nevertheless, this new treatment has gained wide acceptance, especially in Europe, but in North America too, and increasingly, many medical centers are treating half or more of their subarachnoid hemorrhage patients using endovascular techniques. One recent review of this subject published in *Lancet* makes the statement that endovascular treatment is "the treatment of choice" and that surgery is now second. This represents a true paradigm shift that is in the process of occurring.

This shift in the kind of treatment has had another impact: where should patients with intracranial aneurysms be treated? Formerly, when surgery was the only option, most patients were treated at any hospital where a properly trained neurosurgeon could do the procedure. Endovascular technology is normally centralized into high-volume tertiary medical centers. Thus, patients are now often transferred to these centers so that they have the option of whichever treatment (surgical vs. endovascular) best suits their particular situation. Two other advantages of this strategy are that (1) the more procedures done, the better the individuals get at doing them, and (2) there is better neurocritical care offered. Essentially, this is just another example of why stroke centers work.

AVM AND OTHER VASCULAR ABNORMALITIES

AVM stands for arteriovenous malformation. This means that there is a tangle of abnormal blood vessels directly connecting an artery to a vein without the usual orderly progression of a capillary bed in between. This can happen anywhere in the body, but here we are referring just to brain AVMs. Because of this direct connection, arterial blood under high pressure flows directly into veins that are not equipped to handle this kind of pressure. So patients with AVMs may have a hemorrhagic stroke, if blood escapes into the brain tissue. This often happens in relatively young people, ages twenty to forty.

There are three types of treatment available for these patients: surgery, radiation, and endovascular solutions. Because of this, patients with AVM are best treated in a specialized stroke center where all of these modalities are available, so that the best specific treatment (or combination of them) can be selected.

Like with most situations in medicine in which more than one treatment is possible, there are advantages and disadvantages of each kind of therapy. For example, an advantage of surgery is that the cure is immediate, but a disadvantage is that normal brain tissue may be injured at surgery, leaving serious neurological disability. The advantage of radiation is that there is no direct (surgical) trauma to the area; however, it may take many months to experience the positive effects of radiation.

Recently, some endovascular techniques have been used to infuse rapidly setting glue into the AVM to obliterate it. This endovascular obliteration may be only partial; therefore, sometimes combinations of treatments are used. For example, some of the AVM is reduced in size using endovascular treatments in the hope of making surgery better tolerated. Similarly, radiation is sometimes used with surgery or endovascular therapy. Interestingly, some AVM patients also have aneurysms, so a combined treatment approach may be required. Finally, there are different, less common kinds of vascular malformations that require various combinations of these treatments.

VENOUS SINUS THROMBOSIS

Venous sinus thrombosis is unique in the range of ICH because it is the venous rather than the arterial side of the circulation that is involved. The veins that drain blood from the brain back to the heart coalesce into venous sinuses, or pools of venous blood. Sometimes, the blood within either the veins, or more commonly within the sinuses, will clot. As we learned about earlier, this generally occurs in patients who have a reason to make their blood hypercoagulable.

When the blood clots, it interferes with the normal flow of blood back to the heart. Pressure can build up, and this can result in bleeding. This in turn can lead to destruction of brain tissue—stroke—in unusual locations that do not match with specific arterial territories. Seizures are also much more common in venous sinus thrombosis. Another reason that this is an unusual situation in the area of hemorrhagic stroke is that, despite the fact that there is blood in the brain, unbelievably, heparin, a potent blood thinner, is given.

This seems counterintuitive, but because the underlying process is one of clotting, the underlying treatment is to thin the clot. Doctors will administer intravenous heparin in this tricky situation. If the amount of clot is extensive, interventionalist physicians will thread a catheter to the area of the clot and inject local tPA to dissolve the clot. Other times, the interventionalist will thread a catheter that mechanically tries to break up the clot. The ultimate goal of all of these therapies is to relieve the venous obstruction and thereby restore normal venous flow.

ARTERIAL DISSECTION

Arteries in the body have three layers, and sometimes blood will push through the innermost layer (the one closest to the inside) and peel apart the middle and/or the outer layers from the inner one (see Figure 7.5). This is called an arterial dissection. The blood within the wall of the artery takes up space and can push into the lumen and reduce the size of the original artery, causing reduced flow. Additionally, all this activity in the arterial wall sometimes induces clot to form. Arterial dissections can then rupture and lead to a hemorrhage, just as in the case of actress Sharon Stone.

Both the vertebral and the carotid arteries can dissect. Arterial dissections sometimes result in clot formation within the vessel, which results in an ischemic stroke. Other times, the arterial wall weakens, which results in a

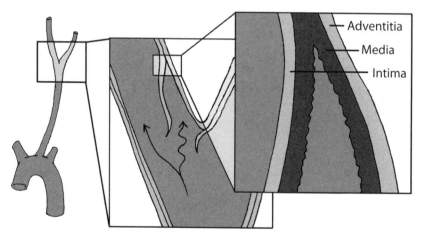

Adventitia
Media
Intima

Figure 7.5. An arterial dissection. The arrows in the middle inset show the blood flowing into the carotid artery. The straight arrow on the left shows blood following the normal course, but the blood on the right (curvy arrow) has dissected into the layers of the artery. The blown-up inset (to the right) shows the three layers of the carotid artery and how the blood has "dissected" between them, splitting the layers and weakening the wall. If the dissection is large, it can close off the vessel and cause an ischemic stroke. If it weakens the outer layer too much, it can rupture and cause a hemorrhagic stroke. Dissections can occur in either the carotid or the vertebral arteries.

hemorrhagic stroke. In the first case, heparin is used. If hemorrhage predominates, then once again, the interventionalist will place a catheter in the area of the dissection and deploy a stent. This will prevent the dissected area from spreading.

VASCULITIS

Occasionally, arteries in the body can get either inflamed or, rarely, infected by a microorganism. In the case of inflammation, the term used to describe inflammation of a blood vessel is "vasculitis." This is fairly uncommon in the cerebral circulation. Like arterial dissection, inflammation can lead

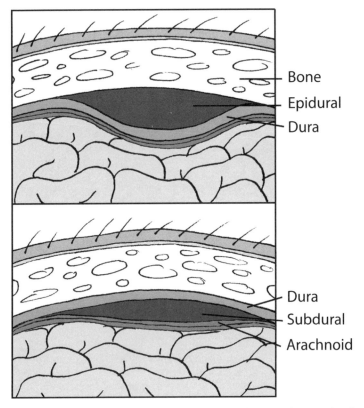

Figure 7.6. The location of the blood (darkest gray area) as it relates to the dura, the brain, and the skull. Epidural hemorrhages (hematomas) are just beneath the skull bone and are usually from a torn artery. Subdural hemorrhages (hematomas) are beneath the dura but outside the arachnoid membrane and are usually attributable to torn veins.

to clotting or bleeding, depending on how much damage occurs in the blood vessel. Cerebral vasculitis is usually treated with potent anti-inflammatory drugs called steroids, usually prednisone.

SUBDURAL AND EPIDURAL HEMORRHAGE

These two entities are not, strictly speaking, hemorrhagic strokes, but they are worth mentioning because they are kinds of ICH and they can present like a hemorrhagic stroke. Recall that the outer and thickest layer of the meninges is called the dura mater. Figure 7.6 shows the relationship of the dura to the brain and shows the locations of subdural hemorrhage (or hematoma) and epidural hemorrhage (or hematoma). The epidural hematoma is outside of the dura and lies next to the skull itself, and the subdural hematoma lies beneath the dura and adjacent to the subarachnoid membrane of the meninges.

The blood collection in either location can cause pressure on the adjacent brain and act just like a stroke. The CT scan will show evidence of blood. The treatment of these two entities is primarily surgical. The neurosurgeon will open the skull, remove the blood clot, and stop the source of the bleeding. These two problems are generally associated with head trauma, but, for subdural hematoma, the trauma can be quite trivial, especially in elderly patients.

Both of these problems are, to some extent, time sensitive and need to be treated rapidly. However, now that doctors are getting more CT scans in elderly patients who fall, they are finding out that many patients have very small clots that will reabsorb with time and will not require surgery. Last, patients who are taking blood thinners may need treatment for the underlying coagulopathy as discussed above.

8

Long-Term Outcomes

We have discussed the acute treatment of stroke and those events that occur in the hospital and over the first days to weeks after the event. These patients are in hospitals where all of the day-to-day activities are managed for the patient. If they need a bath, a healthcare worker can bathe them. If they need to be fed, someone can literally spoon-feed them. If they are unable to take anything by mouth, they can be fed by a tube in the nose or intravenously. If they need assistance in getting from the bed to a chair, help is available.

However, at some point, the patient leaves the hospital. Some go home. Some go to a rehabilitation facility, either short term or long term. And some patients die. There are essentially only three possibilities. A patient can end up normal or near normal. A patient can have enough disability so that they cannot live independently. And a patient can die.

The percentage of each category is a bit different depending on the kind of stroke, the age of the patient, and what kind of condition they were in before the stroke. We will discuss mortality last. However, it is important to consider the philosophic notion that death might not be the worst possibility. In fact, in one study in which people were asked which outcome they most feared, many of them feared paralysis or the inability to speak far more than they feared death.

Let's think about stroke outcomes in terms of the first hour of your day. You wake up in the morning to go to school or work. For many of us, we need an alarm clock to help us. For that, you need to hear the alarm and then, for most alarms, the ability to turn it off. This requires rolling over, finding the clock (partly localizing it by hearing and partly seeing it with your eyes), and having the fine motor coordination to hit the "off" button.

You then get out of bed by using your arms to prop yourself up. Next, you swing your legs off the bed until your feet can reach the floor and then you finally stand up. You then walk to the bathroom to wash your face or shower, brush your teeth, and comb your hair. Each of these activities requires a considerable amount of fine motor coordination. Of course just walking to the bathroom requires strength and an intact cerebellum as well as intact parts of the brainstem.

Next you get dressed. Putting your underwear on requires being able to lift your legs in a coordinated manner, high enough and accurately enough to slip your foot into the opening for the leg, and then pulling them up to your waist. To put pants on, you have to repeat this, but it requires a bit more coordination as the foot tunnels through the pant leg. As for putting on a shirt, you have to be able to lift your arms high enough to slip them into the sleeves and then button the buttons. Think for just a moment about this task. It requires very fine motor coordination that is not always so easy. So too does zipping a zipper, and, depending on what kind of shoes you are wearing, you might need to tie the shoelaces or buckle some buckles. Even if you choose shoes that do not have some kind of fastening device, you still need to get your feet in the shoes.

If you are wearing a belt, you must pass the belt through the belt loops of the pants and then buckle it. You might have almost-invisible contact lenses to delicately put in each eye or want to apply makeup, which takes a steady hand. You then go to have something for breakfast. Even assuming someone is doing the food preparation, you still need to lift the cup of beverage to your mouth and be able to swallow it. Again, this requires a certain degree of fine motor coordination, not to mention that the mouth and throat muscles must be working normally for smooth swallowing to occur (and to avoid aspiration of food or drink into the lungs). You might have to butter a piece of toast, or cut a bite from an omelet, or bring a spoonful of cereal to your mouth. During this time, you may be having a conversation with your family that requires the ability to form language in your brain and then to speak. Your mouth must be working normally. The language center in your left cerebral hemisphere must be intact.

You pick up your textbooks, and it is an unusual student who is not lifting up several pounds of books, placing them into a knapsack or book bag. This requires strength and coordination. You might then meet some friends to wait for a bus or begin to walk to school or work. In either case, you need to do some walking and probably negotiate some stairs to get from where you start to wherever you end up.

We could go through this exercise for your whole day or a whole week but just thinking about the first hour gives you the picture. Almost everything we do, although we're not conscious of all the neurological background functions, requires every portion of our brains to be intact and working well for us to get through a day.

Doctors have devised various scales to measure our ability to function. The NIH stroke scale, which we discussed earlier, is one crude measure. It is essentially a measure of the physical examination, but it really doesn't tell us much about how a given person can function over the course of a day. Therefore, other scales were developed to try to better measure this.

Three major scales are used. These are the Barthel index (see Table 8.1), the Glasgow outcome score (see Table 8.2), and the modified Rankin scale (see Table 8.3). The first scale, the Barthel index, is the most detailed. It was

Table 8.1.
Barthel Index

Feeding
10   Independent; feeds self from tray or table; accomplishes feeding in reasonable time
5   Assistance necessary with cutting food, etc.
0   Cannot meet criteria

Moving (from wheelchair to bed and return)
15   Independent in all phases of this activity
10   Minimal help needed or patient needs to be reminded or supervised for safety of one or more parts of this activity
5   Patient can come to sitting position without help of second person but needs to be lifted out of bed and assisted with transfers
0   Cannot meet criteria

Personal toilet
5   Can wash hands, face; combs hair, cleans teeth; can shave (males) or apply makeup (females) without assistance; females need not brush or style hair
0   Cannot meet criteria

Getting on and off toilet
10   Able to get on and off toilet, fastens/unfastens clothes, can use toilet paper without assistance; may use wall bar or other support if needed; if bedpan necessary, patient can place it on chair, empty, and clean it
5   Needs help because of imbalance or other problems with clothes or toilet paper
0   Cannot meet criteria

Bathing self
5   May use bathtub, shower, or sponge bath; patient must be able to perform all functions without another person being present
0   Cannot meet criteria

(continued)

Table 8.1.
(Continued)

Walking on level surface

15   Patient can walk at least 50 yards without assistance or supervision; may use braces, prostheses, crutches, canes, or walkerette but not a rolling walker; must be able to lock/unlock braces, assume standing or seated position, get mechanical aids into position for use and dispose of them when seated (putting on and off braces should be scored under dressing)

10   Assistance needed to perform above activities but can walk 50 yards with little help

0   Cannot meet criteria

Propelling a wheelchair

      Do not score this item if patient gets score for walking

5   Patient cannot ambulate but can propel wheelchair independently; can go around corners, turn around, maneuver chair to table, bed, toilet, etc. Must be able to push chair 50 yards

0   Cannot meet criteria

Ascending and descending stairs

10   Able to go up and down flight of stairs safely without supervision using canes, handrails, or crutches when needed and can carry these items as ascending/descending

5   Needs help with or supervision of any of the above items

0   Cannot meet criteria

Dressing/undressing

10   Able to put on, fasten, and remove all clothing; ties shoelaces unless necessary adaptations are used; activity includes fastening braces when prescribed; suspenders, loafer shoes and dresses opening in the front may be used when necessary

5   Needs help putting on, fastening, or removing clothing; must accomplish at least half of task alone within reasonable time

0   Cannot meet criteria

Continence of bowels

10   Able to control bowels and have no accidents; can use a suppository or take an enema when necessary (as for spinal cord injury patients who have had bowel training)

5   Needs help in using a suppository or taking an enema or has occasional accidents

0   Cannot meet criteria

Controlling bladder

10   Able to control bladder day and night; spinal injury patients must be able to put on external devices and leg bags independently, clean and empty bag, and must stay dry day and night

5   Occasional accidents occur, cannot wait for bed pan, does not get to toilet in time or needs help with external device

0   Cannot meet criteria

Table 8.2.
The Glasgow Outcome Score

Score	Description
1	Death
2	Persistent vegetative state: patient exhibits no obvious cortical function
3	Severe disability (conscious but disabled): patient depends on others for daily support as a result of mental or physical disability or both
4	Moderate disability (disabled but independent): patient is independent as far as daily life is concerned; the disabilities found include varying degrees of dysphasia, hemiparesis, or ataxia, as well as intellectual and memory deficits and personality changes
5	Good recovery: resumption of normal activities, although there may be minor neurological or psychological deficits

developed more than forty years ago, and it contains all of the elements that we discussed in your first hour of the day: feeding, moving about, personal care items, negotiating stairs, dressing, and bowel and bladder function. Points are given or not, and a normal individual will have a score of 100.

The Glasgow outcome score was developed more than thirty years ago and was initially developed to describe the outcome in patients with head trauma. Because it is a five-point score, it is much less detailed than the Barthel index. It gives a rough idea about how a patient is doing but does not drill down the specific reason why.

The modified Rankin scale is the oldest of all, having first been developed in 1957. Similar to the Glasgow score, the modified Rankin scale is also a less

Table 8.3.
Modified Rankin Scale

Score	Description
0	No symptoms at all
1	No significant disability despite symptoms; able to perform all usual duties and activities
2	Slight disability; unable to perform all previous activities but able to look after own affairs without assistance
3	Moderate disability; requiring some help but able to walk without assistance
4	Moderately severe disability; unable to walk without assistance and unable to attend to own bodily needs without assistance
5	Severe disability; bedridden, incontinent, and requiring constant nursing care and attention
6	Dead

detailed measure, being a six-point score. Although all of these outcome scales are important, the modified Rankin scale is the one that the majority of neurologists use most often. It is also the one that is most commonly used by researchers studying stroke treatments. This one is worth understanding to appreciate the results of this research.

Look at the difference between a Rankin 1 and 2. Some researchers have used a modified Rankin of 0 or 1 to indicate an "excellent" outcome, whereas others have used a breakpoint of 0–2 to indicate "good" outcome or "independent" living. Although a 0, 1, or 2 indicates a fairly good outcome, there is a big difference between a modified Rankin 1 and a 2. Both can live independently, but those patients who are classified as a Rankin 1 can perform all previous activities, whereas those who are Rankin 2 will need help with such things as dressing or perhaps with cooking their food.

As you can see from Table 8.3, increasing Rankin scores are associated with decreasing ability to function independently. As mentioned above, some people would prefer to die from a large stroke (Rankin 6) than be severely disabled (Rankin 4 or 5).

However, there is another side to the disability that is associated with stroke, and this is the emotional and societal cost of stroke, both domestically and internationally. For the most part, stroke patients are older, and the loss of independence is an enormous psychological loss. It marks the reversal of a lifelong relationship with friends, family, work, and hobbies. Someone who was always the leader of a family is now in need of help from their children. Those with jobs may no longer be able to work, or may not be able to drive themselves, or take public transportation to work. A person who enjoys bird watching or boating may no longer be able to have the balance or the stamina to continue with these activities.

There are downstream economic and psychiatric effects of stroke. The financial costs can be vast. There are the direct costs such as the hospital bills and the doctor fees for follow-up visits. Indirect costs would include the loss of productivity that the patient would have been able to do if he had not been affected by a stroke. Another example would be the lost work time for a relative taking a day off to drive their father to a doctor's appointment. Remember that these costs accrue over time. A patient who has a stroke at age fifty has decades to come, during which costs will accumulate.

An Australian study using data from 1997 found that the total lifetime costs were greater for ischemic stroke (the equivalent of US $710 million) and less for ICH (US $253 million). The average cost per case (during just the first year) was greatest for total anterior circulation infarction at approximately $25,000.

A U.S. study, using numbers from Medicare databases, showed that the first four years of stroke care averaged $48,000 for subarachnoid hemorrhage patients, $38,000 for ICH patients, and $39,000 for ischemic stroke patients. Each of these figures is per patient. The authors of this study also concluded that "with the expected increase in the elderly population over the coming decades, these results emphasize the need for effective preventive and acute medical care."

The annual cost of care for a single individual living in a nursing home after a stroke ranges from $54,000 to $72,000, depending on the level of care needed and the facilities. Approximately 20 percent of patients who have suffered a stroke will require institutional care within three months of their event.

These studies are all based on certain assumptions, and the figures that they calculate are somewhat different from one another. However, they all come to the same conclusion, which is that stroke care for the entire population is very expensive.

There are pharmacy costs as well. Medications to prevent recurrent strokes cost money, and these drugs usually must be taken every day, and the high-tech endovascular interventions that were discussed in the chapters on treatment are extraordinarily expensive. Recall that, for patients with subarachnoid hemorrhage from a ruptured aneurysm, the aneurysm can be treated by endovascular coiling or open surgical clipping. Patients whose aneurysms are clipped must stay in the ICU longer and will have costly surgeons' fees, but the costs of the coils themselves are so high that coiling was actually more expensive than clipping in one European study.

So, not only is the population getting older (which means that more patients will suffer from strokes), but the cost of treating each patient is rising, both because of inflation in general and because newer, often better techniques are generally more expensive than older, lower-tech treatments.

In 1997, the total cost of stroke in the United States was estimated to be about $41 billion. A more recent U.S. study estimated that the total cost of all stroke care in the United States, in 2005, added up to approximately $57 billion. This figure only relates to the United States, and, although U.S. healthcare is generally more expensive than in other countries, many other countries, especially developed countries, also spend a lot of money on stroke care.

Add to that the emotional toll to both patients and families. Depression after a stroke is very common. Even patients who have had a good outcome following a stroke may experience anxiety and depression about having a recurrent event. Patients who are left dependent on others are often frustrated and suffer guilt because of the burden they have placed on loved ones.

Although some people would rather die than be severely disabled, many people do not feel this way. For this reason alone, mortality is still an important measure of the "cost" of stroke. Second, mortality is an important standard measure of outcome for any serious disease. What is the mortality of stroke?

Mortality rate is generally computed as the percentage of patients who die within ninety days of their stroke. For acute ischemic stroke, the mortality rate ranges from roughly 10 to 20 percent. For ICH, the mortality rate is 40–50 percent, and, for subarachnoid hemorrhage, mortality approaches 50 percent. Of course the cost of emotional, societal, and personal factors can never be properly measured, but it is safe to say that these costs are enormous.

It may seem perfectly obvious, but treatment affects outcomes. Mortality rates have dropped over the past thirty to forty years in the United States. Why is this? Much of it derives from better overall care: better hypertension treatment, improved diet, more attention to cholesterol-lowering therapy, and far better diabetes control. As well, there is gradually increasing knowledge among the general population about the symptoms of stroke, so patients often show up sooner than they did twenty years ago. This opens up more treatment options for the doctor, and starting medical care sooner can prevent some of the complications before they have time to develop.

Another reason for the decrease is better acute treatments, especially for treating patients who have had TIA or minor stroke. These treatments are aimed at preventing another stroke, which might have far worse consequences. Increasing use of stroke centers, which put more focus on preventative measures such as early mobilization (to prevent blood clots in the legs) and swallowing (to prevent aspiration of food or liquids into the lungs), has been shown to improve clinical outcomes. In addition, the use of standardized orders in these patients helps to reduce the likelihood of forgetting to dispense a certain medication or treatment.

Providing standardized treatments is important. Not starting physical therapy could leave a patient at risk of falling, and a fall in an elderly patient often results in a wrist fracture, a broken hip, or a head injury. Even the most minor of the three, a wrist fracture, that requires a cast and a sling can seriously affect a person's ability to take care of their daily needs. Hip fractures are even more devastating because they require surgery to repair, and, unfortunately, surgery in the elderly opens the door to still more problems. Obviously, a head injury complicating a stroke can lead to far worse neurological outcomes.

Despite all of these advances, a great deal still needs to be accomplished to improve the outcomes of stroke patients even more.

9

Preventing Stroke

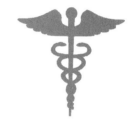

From the previous few chapters, several points should be quite obvious. First, treating stroke is extremely resource intensive on many levels. Most of the newer treatments are expensive. Huge amounts of caregivers' time and specialized expertise, not to mention a lot of money, are spent taking care of stroke patients. This is time and money that, if a stroke could be prevented, could be spent on something else. The enormous personal, emotional, and social burden to society is a cost that is much harder to measure but easy to understand. Caring for a stroke patient who cannot speak, and cannot live independently, and who might live for another ten years in some type of chronic-care institution depletes many resources on all of these levels.

From the last chapter, it is also obvious that, although we are doing better with stroke care, there is a long way to go, and many of the long-term outcomes are not favorable. Considering the huge worldwide stroke burden and the aging population, one can see that stroke imparts an enormous negative impact on society that will only increase in magnitude in coming years.

For all of these reasons, it should be clear that preventing a stroke is far preferable to treating a stroke, and many of the risk factors that were discussed in Chapter 2 are modifiable or treatable. Stroke prevention focuses on doing

whatever measures are possible to change those modifiable risk factors to minimize the likelihood of a stroke in the first place.

One distinction that is usually made is that of "primary" stroke prevention
vs. "secondary" stroke prevention. Primary stroke prevention means preventing a stroke before it ever occurs. Secondary prevention means preventing a
stroke in a patient who has already had either a stroke or a TIA. Many measures, such as treating high blood pressure and smoking cessation, are important
for both primary and secondary prevention. The same applies to treating a
patient with a PFO or an arterial dissection. In this book, we will not highlight this distinction between primary and secondary prevention here. We will
discuss secondary stroke prevention after a TIA in the next chapter.

The World Health Organization estimates that 75 percent of strokes in
middle-aged people can be attributed to an unfavorable risk factor profile. As
we discussed in Chapter 2, some risk factors cannot be modified: age, race, sex,
family history, and genetic predisposition. Although these cannot change, people with unmodifiable high risk factors often also have acquired risk factors
that are treatable. It is important that doctors focus, at least, on changing the
risks that can be changed. This is helpful because such a large percentage of
patients with stroke do have modifiable risk factors, and intervening on these
can have a huge impact in terms of both primary and secondary prevention.

In this chapter, we will focus on various specific preventative strategies for
both ischemic and hemorrhagic strokes. This is such an important topic that
the AHA published a nearly forty-page document on stroke prevention in
2006, and all of its clinical guidelines focus on disease prevention.

LIFESTYLE MODIFICATIONS

There are some elements of stroke prevention that are easier said than
done. Issues that are deeply embedded in our culture, things such as smoking,
alcohol consumption, dietary issues, and exercise, are things that are difficult
to get people to change. For example, eating a diet rich in fruits and vegetables and low in animal fats has been associated with lower blood pressure, but
getting patients to change their diets is not an easy thing to accomplish. In
modern times, people work more and spend less time on food preparation. In
general, eating a healthy diet takes more thought (to buy fresh ingredients)
and a great deal more time (to prepare them). Increasingly, people are buying
and eating more processed foods and pre-prepared foods. As a general rule,
these foods are less healthy than fresh food because of processing and food
additives. Also, they are often heavy in unhealthy fats. Europeans tend to use
olive oil instead of animal-based fats such as butter, which Americans often

use. Also, their diet traditionally has been richer in fruits and vegetables. In recent years, this healthier diet has been termed The Mediterranean Diet.

Obesity is becoming epidemic in the United States. The relationship of obesity to stroke is complicated, because obesity is also associated with high blood pressure, diabetes, and elevated cholesterol, all stroke risk factors in their own right. That said, at least in men, obesity by itself seems to be a risk, especially when the body fat is concentrated around the abdomen. Although no study has specifically shown that weight loss reduces the risk of stroke, the AHA recommends that overweight individuals undergo weight reduction by diet, exercise, and behavior modification. Recently, studies have shown that weight is a significant factor in cancer as well as heart disease; thus, it would not be surprising if there is also a link between obesity or an unhealthy diet and stroke.

Smoking cigarettes is a risk factor for ischemic stroke and subarachnoid hemorrhage. This is true in both sexes, in all racial and ethnic groups, and across the age spectrum. One large study found that smokers had twice the risk of stroke as nonsmokers. The likely mechanism for this is that smoking affects the blood vessels. Patients who quit smoking seem to lose the excess risk imparted by their previous smoking after about five years. It is important to note that second-hand smoking (that is, being exposed to someone else's cigarette smoke) also increases stroke risk, so one person's quitting can also benefit others in the same household.

Of course there are many other health benefits to smoke avoidance. Smoking contributes to chronic lung disease such as bronchitis and emphysema. It is a major risk for lung cancer. Smokers have higher heart attack rates and a disease of the other arteries of the body called peripheral artery disease. Both of these last two are attributable to the effects of smoking on atherosclerosis.

There are many ways to help patients stop smoking, including many nicotine-containing products that help to treat the pharmacological tobacco dependence. There are also counseling and oral smoking cessation medications to be tried. Some people have luck with acupuncture, and many others have success stopping on their own. Because smoking is to some extent a nicotine addiction, treating it as an addiction with all of these modalities can help a person stop smoking.

Although the effect of alcohol on stroke risk is not entirely clear, there is fairly good evidence that heavy or chronic drinking increases the risk for stroke. Recent binge drinking is a risk factor for subarachnoid hemorrhage. At the same time, the relationship between ischemic stroke and alcohol consumption is more complicated. In fact, light to moderate alcohol consumption may actually reduce the risk of ischemic stroke.

When investigators have analyzed pooled data from many different studies that have tried to sort out this relationship, they found that heavy drinking (defined as more than five drinks per day) had an increased risk of stroke, but patients who drank one to two drinks per day actually had a reduced risk. In this study, they defined one drink as a twelve-ounce beer, a four-ounce glass of wine, or a cocktail with one and a half ounces of liquor. The mechanism of this lowered risk may be an increase in "good" cholesterol or changes in blood coagulation that have been associated with alcohol consumption. Heavy drinking, of course, can result in health problems such as liver disease, gastrointestinal bleeding, and others that are independent of their effects on stroke.

Exercise and increased physical activity have many benefits to the body, especially the cardiovascular system. Reviews of medical literature suggest that highly active individuals have a lower risk than those with low levels of activity. Physical activity can help to reduce body weight and blood pressure, decrease the tendency to become diabetic, and can result in beneficial effects on blood vessels. Moderate activity may reduce the risk of stroke by 20 percent, and heavy physical activity reduces the risk by nearly 30 percent. The AHA guideline on stroke prevention recommends at least thirty minutes of moderate intensity physical activity most days of the week. Again, as with smoking cessation and avoiding heavy alcohol consumption, there are innumerable health benefits to physical activity beyond stroke prevention. Furthermore, none of them require any life-long medications or other expensive treatments.

HYPERTENSION (HIGH BLOOD PRESSURE)

Approximately fifty million Americans have high blood pressure, and this constitutes a risk for both ischemic and hemorrhagic stroke. For the former, the higher the blood pressure, the higher the risk of stroke. Medical studies are very clear that, by reducing high blood pressure, 30–40 percent of that risk is lowered. Although the risk of both first-ever and secondary strokes can be reduced by lowering a high blood pressure, there is less evidence in regard to lowering blood pressure for secondary prevention. Many of these studies have studied a combination of three different endpoints: heart attack, stroke, and death of any cause.

One European study tried to quantify how much lower the blood pressure needed to be to reduce the risk of stroke. They enrolled 5,000 patients over sixty years of age. They compared a kind of drug called a calcium channel blocker (to which could be added another kind of drug called an "angiotensin-converting enzyme inhibitor") with placebo. The amount of blood pressure reduction, which occurred rapidly, was an average of 23/7 (twenty-three points on the systolic and seven points off the diastolic values). At four years, there was a 42 percent reduction in both fatal and nonfatal stroke. They concluded that even a modest reduction in blood pressure can result in a marked reduction in stroke risk.

Because most patients with high blood pressure do not have symptoms, it is very important that doctors explain the purpose and importance of the medications because the side effects of medications can start right away, but the therapeutic effects (lowered blood pressure to prevent a stroke or heart attack) are never "visible" to the patient.

Other trials of different anti-hypertensive drugs have produced similar results. It seems that lowering the blood pressure, no matter by what means, is the underlying mechanism of decreasing later strokes and other vascular events. There is no particular medication or class of medication that is needed. Furthermore, lowering blood pressure by nonpharmacologic means, such as weight reduction, dietary changes, exercise, smoking cessation, and others, will also help reduce the risk of subsequent stroke. The AHA guidelines call for modest reductions (average of 10/5) in blood pressure of patients who have already had strokes or TIA. Because other guidelines have been gradually aiming toward lower and lower target blood pressure, the AHA guidelines call for this treatment even in patients without a previous history of hypertension. Furthermore, although the document does not set a specific target blood pressure, it does reference a definition of "normal" of less than 120/80.

DIABETES

Diabetes is a common problem that affects 8 percent of the adult population and is a worldwide problem. In studies of both TIA patients and the general population, diabetes has been identified as a risk factor for ischemic stroke. In patients who have already had a stroke, diabetes is correlated with recurrent strokes. Diabetes is a disease of carbohydrate or sugar metabolism, and the cardinal feature is reduced insulin function leading to high levels of blood sugar. The normal level of blood sugar when a person is fasting is from 60 to 100 mg/dl of blood. The threshold for diagnosing diabetes is greater than 126 mg/dl. When a diabetic is acutely ill, they will sometimes come to an ED with a blood sugar of 600 or 700 mg/dl.

Diabetes affects the small and large blood vessels, heart, brain, eyes, peripheral nerves, and kidneys, so as with smoking cigarettes and high blood pressure, treating diabetes has a positive health effect well beyond just stroke prevention. Many years ago, doctors gave insulin, the hormone that lowers blood sugar, to reduce high blood sugars. However, because patients could be harmed if the blood sugar fell too far, they did not try to achieve too low of a target blood sugar. During this era, patients did not have access to small portable measuring devices, and the types of insulin and other medications for treating diabetes were limited.

Over the past twenty years or so, doctors who treat diabetes have increasingly focused on exact blood sugar control (tight glycemic control), attempting to maintain normal or near-normal levels. Some diabetic patients will inject insulin two, three, or even four times per day and check their blood sugar the same number of times to maintain this specific glycemic control. So some of the reason that patients maintain tight control is that they have the tools to do so, but, in addition, studies over the past few decades strongly suggest that close glycemic control reduces the vascular complications of diabetes. Doctors measure how "tight" the glycemic control is by measuring hemoglobin A1C levels.

When the blood sugar is high for long periods of time, it binds to the hemoglobin in the blood. Unlike blood sugar, hemoglobin levels do not change rapidly. This hemoglobin with the bound sugar is called "glycosylated" hemoglobin, or hemoglobin A1C. Doctors can follow the hemoglobin A1C level to get a sort of rolling average of how a patient's blood sugar has been doing for the past few weeks. Doctors try to keep the percentage of hemoglobin A1C below 7 percent. Last, with respect to diabetes, all of the lifestyle modifications such as smoking cessation, exercise, and alcohol reduction help to improve the blood sugar control.

Many of the studies on diabetes control also included other interventions, such as blood pressure treatment and lowering of blood lipid levels. The following three conditions, hypertension, elevated lipids, and diabetes, in combination all lead to worse effects on the blood vessels of the body than any one of them in isolation. Because of this, in diabetic patients, doctors have started using lower targets for blood pressure control or lipid levels than in nondiabetic patients, so the presence of diabetes also affects the approach to other stroke risk factors.

Therefore, official recommendations are that doctors try to more rigorously control elevated blood pressure and blood lipids. As well, some specific kinds of medications seem to be particularly effective in reducing the kidney complications of diabetes. A detailed discussion of these agents is beyond the scope of this chapter. However, for the interested reader, they are called angiotensin-converting enzyme inhibitors and angiotensin receptor blockers.

BLOOD LIPIDS

Recall from Chapter 2 that cholesterol is a fatty substance in the blood that is a critical component of cells in the body but that, in high levels, is a risk factor for blockages in large arteries. There are different subtypes of cholesterol that are based on their molecular structure. The two most important ones relevant to this topic are low-density lipoprotein (LDL) and high-density lipoprotein (HDL) cholesterol. As mentioned earlier in the book, LDL cholesterol is also referred to as "bad" cholesterol and HDL as "good" cholesterol.

Higher levels of LDL are associated with higher risk of stroke (and other vascular disease such as heart attack). Interestingly, higher levels of HDL seem to be protective and are desirable, hence the term "good" cholesterol. In general, higher levels of triglycerides, another fatty substance in the blood, are associated with higher risk of stroke.

Patients with elevated LDL can be risk stratified into different groups. In low-risk individuals, defined as patients having no more than one vascular risk factor, the recommended goals are to get the level of LDL below 160 mg/dl. Patients with two or more risk factors should try to get their LDL below 130 mg/dl. In diabetics and other higher-risk patients, the goal is to treat the LDL until it is below 100 mg/dl. Last, newer information suggests that there is a fourth category of patients with a very high risk of stroke whose target LDL levels should be less than 70 mg/dl!

The elements that are used in determining this level of risk show how inter-related the situation is. Diabetes, ongoing smoking, and high blood pressure care were certainly factored in. So were the presence of other vascular problems such as established coronary atherosclerosis and a person's overall physical condition and lifestyle. Much of the data for these recommendations come not only from studying stroke patients but from studying cardiac patients as well.

There is a class of drug that is called "statins." This group of medications, of which there are at least six, lowers LDL cholesterol levels. Statins inhibit an enzyme called 3-hydroxy-3-methyl-glutaryl-coenzyme A, which controls the rate of cholesterol production in the body. This decreases the production of cholesterol and also increases the liver's ability to remove the LDL cholesterol already in the blood.

Studies using statins have reported 20–60 percent lower LDL cholesterol levels in patients on these drugs. As an additional benefit, statins also produce a modest increase in HDL cholesterol and reduce elevated triglyceride levels. Studies also have begun to show that there may be some form of risk reduction from statins that is independent of the cholesterol-lowering mechanism.

Analysis of many different clinical trials testing statin drugs showed a 21 percent risk reduction in stroke, including a slight reduction in fatal strokes. The statin effect was closely associated with the reduction in LDL cholesterol, which the investigators concluded accounted for 34–80 percent of the observed benefit. Remarkably, each 10 percent reduction in LDL cholesterol was estimated to reduce the risk of all strokes by 13 percent.

Extrapolating all of this information, doctors thought that perhaps very aggressive treatment with statins could even further lower risk for stroke and heart attacks, so they began the Stroke Prevention by Aggressive Reduction in Cholesterol Levels (SPARCL) trial. SPARCL was designed to test the effects of statin therapy in nearly 5,000 patients who previously had a stroke or TIA and who had no known cardiovascular disease.

SPARCL showed that using a high-dose statin regimen reduced stroke by 16 percent and major coronary events by 35 percent. However, they also found a very small increase in the incidence of hemorrhagic stroke.

All of this information has led to the AHA's recommendation that "patients with ischemic stroke or TIA presumed to be of an atherosclerotic origin but with no preexisting indications for statins (normal cholesterol, no coexistent coronary artery disease, and no evidence of atherosclerosis) are reasonable candidates for treatment with a statin to reduce the rate of vascular events." This represents an important change because doctors are now treating patients with normal cholesterol levels with statins.

In general, this class of medication is well tolerated, but a very small minority of patients will have a serious complication that results in severe inflammation and destruction of skeletal muscle cells, which can be, on rare occasion, fatal. Usually, the symptoms resolve with discontinuing the statin.

Last, there are some other classes of medications that impact cholesterol levels, such as gemfibrozil and niacin, which to some extent act by increasing HDL cholesterol levels.

ATRIAL FIBRILLATION

As discussed in Chapter 2, atrial fibrillation is the chaotic rhythm of the top chambers of the heart. Because the atria lose the ability to pump in a coordinated manner, clots form, which can then travel to the brain and cause an ischemic stroke. Clinicians have known for decades that patients with atrial fibrillation are at higher risk for stroke. Although the annual risk of stroke in these patients is approximately 3–5 percent, patients can have this rhythm for many years, so the risk is cumulative. In addition, atrial fibrillation is very common, affecting more than two million Americans. Furthermore, the incidence of atrial fibrillation increases with age.

As with elevated blood lipids, stroke risk in atrial fibrillation patients increases greater still if they have other conditions such as hypertension, diabetes, heart failure, and previous stroke or TIA.

Many studies have shown that treating these patients with anticoagulants such as Coumadin reduces this risk. To get a better idea of the magnitude of this reduction, doctors pooled data from five different studies and found a nearly 70 percent risk reduction in patients using Coumadin. Patients on a placebo had a stroke risk of 4.5 percent, whereas those treated with Coumadin had a 1.4 percent stroke rate. Coumadin works as a blood thinner so clot cannot form in the chaotically beating atria of the heart.

However, Coumadin treatment has its challenges. This is a medication with what doctors call a "narrow therapeutic window." This means that the range of the dosage of Coumadin that is effective without producing side effects is very narrow. The effect of the blood thinning of Coumadin is measured with a blood test called the international normalized ratio (INR). A normal person not on Coumadin will have an INR of 1.0; the therapeutic goal for patients on Coumadin is 2.0–3.0. If the INR falls below 2.0, it is much less effective and patients can form clot and are at risk of having a stroke. Conversely, if the INR goes above 3, patients' blood is too thin and they are at risk of bleeding. Recall that one important cause of hemorrhagic stroke is that it is associated with oral anticoagulant therapy, most of the time with Coumadin.

Many things affect the INR, so finding the right dose for a patient can change with time. There is a long list of medications and foods that can change the INR, necessitating a dose adjustment, at least in the short term. For example, when a patient takes an antibiotic for an unrelated infection, their INR can skyrocket. Some drugs will raise the INR, but others will lower it. Patients on Coumadin require close and lifelong monitoring.

Because of all these problems, doctors are always looking for better ways of reducing the risk of clotting in atrial fibrillation patients. They have tested anti-platelet medicines for this condition, but the data for aspirin (compared with placebo) is much weaker than for Coumadin. Doctors are also testing other combinations of anti-platelet medications such as aspirin plus clopidogrel.

Trials comparing Coumadin with aspirin for stroke reduction in atrial fibrillation show that Coumadin is clearly the better drug, so for now, the standard therapy is long-term anticoagulation with Coumadin. Newer medications that are easier to use and monitor are on the horizon and will be discussed in Chapter 11.

Specifically, the AHA guidelines call for anticoagulation with Coumadin that gives an INR of 2–3. For patients who cannot tolerate oral anticoagulants, aspirin is recommended.

OTHER CARDIO-EMBOLIC SOURCES OF CLOT

There are fewer studies that address other causes of clot in the heart such as cardiomyopathy, heart attack, and valvular heart problems. In each of these situations, the main pumping chamber of the heart, the left ventricle, can dilate. Usually, the more it dilates, the worse is the pumping function. This situation of decreased pump function and a dilated ventricle is a setup for sluggish flow, and sluggish flow can lead to clot formation, just as it does in the atrium in atrial fibrillation patients.

There are a number of studies in each of the above situations, but the amount of patients and the quality of those studies are less than those with atrial fibrillation. In post-heart attack patients, doctors will sometimes do an echocardiogram to look for clot in the left ventricle. This test is simple and non-invasive and can accurately see the clots.

In general, although the quality of the evidence is less for all of these other situations that can lead to cardio-embolic stroke compared with that for atrial fibrillation, the guidelines parallel those for atrial fibrillation.

There are three exceptions. The first is emboli that originate from a valve infected in endocarditis. In this situation, because there is active infection, the chance of bleeding is too great to warrant Coumadin. Second, in patients with mitral valve prolapse (an abnormal movement of the mitral valve and the most common form of valvular heart disease in adults), the risk is lower so only aspirin is recommended. Last, in patients who have surgically implanted "prosthetic" valves, the recommended level of INR is higher (2.5–3.5). Prosthetic valves are made from metal and plastic materials and are therefore more likely to produce clot.

ANTI-PLATELET MEDICATIONS

There are no quality data about the use of aspirin or other anti-platelet medicines purely for primary stroke prevention, other than those mentioned in this chapter for some uses such as atrial fibrillation in patients who cannot tolerate full anticoagulation with Coumadin. For patients who have had another manifestation of vascular disease, such as a heart attack, there is evidence that treating with anti-platelet medications will reduce subsequent heart attacks and stroke. This is usually considered secondary prevention of vascular disease but could be construed as primary prevention of stroke. We will discuss this important group of medications in much greater detail in the next chapter, which deals with TIA.

ASYMPTOMATIC CAROTID STENOSIS

In the early 1990s, large clinical trials were done that showed that patients who had a TIA or minor stroke as well as a blocked carotid artery benefited by opening up the artery surgically. In the next chapter, we will discuss in detail the treatment of TIA patients who have blocked carotid arteries. The surgical procedure is called "carotid endarterectomy," to be covered in detail in the next chapter on TIA. We will discuss the endovascular procedures in Chapter 11 on new horizons. In this chapter, we will discuss the use of this procedure only in asymptomatic patients who have never had neurological symptoms from the blockage.

Extrapolating the information from studies in patients with blocked arteries with TIA to patients who have blocked arteries but who do not have neurological symptoms is not necessarily scientifically correct. In this group (of patients without symptoms), the risk of surgery must be balanced against the fact that a given patient may never have symptoms to begin with. But if the patient has no symptoms, how would they know there is a carotid artery blockage in the first place?

When doctors perform a physical examination, they will place the stethoscope over the patient's neck. Many times, if a patient has a carotid artery blocked by cholesterol plaque, the flow of blood is faster through the narrowed segment of the artery. This rapid and turbulent flow makes a noise that is audible with the stethoscope. The term for this is a "bruit," which comes from the French word for noise. When a patient has a bruit, there are a few possible causes, so the doctor will do an ultrasound or an angiogram to prove that it is attributable to a carotid obstruction and to quantify it. If the obstruction is more than 70 percent, what is the best option? One has to balance the risk of surgery in a patient who is feeling perfectly well (causing a stroke) against the benefits of the surgery (preventing a stroke).

One large study of more than 3,000 patients less than seventy-five years old who had asymptomatic carotid stenosis compared patients who were randomized to receive carotid endarterectomy vs. no endarterectomy. This latter group was the "placebo" group, and some of them had surgery after-the-fact, but very few of them. The investigators then followed them for five years. In the group that got surgery, 3 percent had a stroke or death in the first month after surgery. Was there sufficient benefit in the group treated with surgery to balance these postoperative complications?

Even including the early strokes that occurred in the first postoperative month, the difference was a roughly 6 percent stroke risk in the treated group and a 12 percent risk in the nonsurgical group. Importantly, half of the strokes in the nontreated group were fatal or resulted in severe disability. Another important fact is that the patients who did not have surgery were still being treated with anti-platelet medications, anti-hypertensives, and lipid-lowering agents. This means that the surgery was not being compared with "no" therapy but against "best medical management."

However, because the benefit for asymptomatic patients is less, the practice of doing carotid surgery on asymptomatic individuals is a bit controversial compared with using this treatment in patients who have already had a TIA (as we shall see in the next chapter). In the asymptomatic group, it is especially important to have the very best surgeons with the very lowest complications rate.

ELEVATED HOMOCYSTEINE LEVELS

In Chapter 2, we mentioned that high levels of the amino acid homocysteine likely are a risk factor for stroke and heart disease. There is moderately good evidence for this. Although the evidence for treating this condition is less clear, the latest 2006 AHA guidelines for ischemic stroke prevention include a brief section on treatment of patients with elevated homocysteine levels. The recommendation is for patients to eat diets high in folate and vitamin B12 by eating vegetables, fruits, legumes, meats, fish, and fortified grains. Supplementing intake of folate and B12 by pill, such as a multivitamin, may also help reduce the risk of stroke, but it is best to get vitamins via food.

HYPERCOAGULABLE STATES

For the various hypercoagulable states, it is logical that anticoagulation is recommended. The recommendations are a bit vague on the intensity (target level of the INR) and the duration of the anticoagulation, which reflects less quality in the data that underlie the recommendations. Generally, doctors will use the 2–3 range for the INR.

As for patients with sickle cell disease, transfusions and a medication called hydroxyurea are sometimes used to prevent stroke. Anti-platelet medications are also used in this group of patients.

PFO

Recall that patients with PFO have a hole between the upper chambers of the heart, connecting the right atrium with the left atrium. This hole is a remnant of a normal communication that is found in the fetus; it is actually remarkably common. About 20 percent of normal individuals have a PFO. If such a patient develops a clot, then the clot can travel from the right side to the left side and then embolize to the brain or other parts of the body.

In patients with PFO who have had a TIA or previous stroke, doctors recommend anti-platelet therapy to prevent a recurrent event. Doctors will prescribe Coumadin for patients at high risk of forming a clot (such as those with hypercoagulable states).

In exceptional circumstances, a surgeon can close the PFO surgically. This involves obvious risk from the surgery itself. Over time, doctors have developed percutaneous closure devices. Percutaneous means "through the skin." Doctors will thread a catheter into the vein in the groin and guide it to the heart. They then guide the catheter across the hole in the atria. Next, they place a device over the catheter that crosses the hole, and last, they can deploy this closure device that covers and closes the PFO. These latter solutions would only be used after a patient has had at least one or possibly even two strokes. Because PFO is a relatively common condition in normal individuals, the doctor will want to be sure that the PFO and the stroke are related in a given patient.

INTRACRANIAL ANEURYSM

Regarding subarachnoid hemorrhage, there are three potential ways to prevent the stroke. The first would be to prevent the aneurysm from forming in the first place, but, because doctors do not understand why aneurysms develop, this strategy remains one that cannot be implemented at the present time. The second is to focus on the factors that are associated with increased risk of rupture such as cigarette smoking, hypertension, and heavy alcohol use. The recommendations here are no different from those for ischemic stroke: stop smoking, reduce heavy alcohol use, and treat the high blood pressure.

The major preventative strategy, however, is finding and treating unruptured aneurysms. Many years ago, if an aneurysm was discovered as a surprise finding on an angiogram done for some other reason, the patient would be referred to a neurosurgeon, who would usually recommend surgical clipping. Over the past several years, several developments have impacted this traditional approach.

The first is the fact that many more patients are having brain imaging, often with vascular imaging, so the frequency of patients with incidentally discovered brain aneurysms is increasing. We have known for years that about 2–6 percent of the general population have aneurysms. At the same time, we know that the vast majority of these do not rupture.

The second factor involves the size of the individual aneurysm. This realization emerged from a large study called the International Study of Unruptured Intracranial Aneurysms (ISUIA) that was performed over the last fifteen years. The first part of this study was published in 1998, and a second publication came out in 2003. This study tried to distinguish two groups of patients with aneurysms: those with low (or no) risk of rupture over time and those who were at higher risk of rupture.

One of the most important factors that affect the risk of rupture in this study is aneurysm size. Incidental aneurysms less than 1 cm had a very low risk of rupture, less than 0.05 percent per year. Larger aneurysms had higher rates of rupture. Also, aneurysms in the posterior circulation were more likely to rupture than those in the anterior circulation. Additional work has shown that less than 7 mm should be the cutoff size for aneurysms less likely to rupture. Other factors include gender (females more likely to rupture than males) and ethnicity (patients from Finland and Japan seem to have higher risk that those from other countries).

This risk of rupture must be balanced against the risk of treatment. Up until ten years ago, this meant the risk of neurosurgery, especially in the ISUIA trial that recruited patients before the shift to endovascular treatment. Outcomes of treatment showed that the rate of death or major disability was significant. Remember that these are patients who feel completely normal before the treatment. This is different from subarachnoid hemorrhage patients whose aneurysms have already ruptured. Any problems resulting from the treatment (surgery in most cases) was directly attributable to the surgery and not the aneurysm.

In the ISUIA study, they found that, for patients less than forty-five years of age, the rate of death or disability was about 6 percent, the rate for patients aged forty-five to sixty-five was 14 percent, and the rate for patients older than sixty-five was 32 percent. However, other subsequent studies have found much lower rates of problems related to therapy, and, as endovascular treatments become increasingly the first line of treatment, the level of risk will fall even lower.

Additional factors that doctors must consider are a patient's age as well as other diseases that they may harbor. For example, a forty-year-old healthy individual is at a much lower risk from treatment and also has a much longer period of time over which their aneurysm could rupture. In this situation, fixing the aneurysm would make sense: low risk and high gain. Contrast that situation with a sixty-five-year-old person with lung cancer. Their risk of treatment is higher and their period of risk of rupture is much shorter. In this situation, the best course of action may be to do nothing because of a high risk and a much lower gain.

When should patients undergo screening for aneurysms? Should doctors actively search for aneurysms so that they can fix them before they rupture? Screening the general population makes no sense at all because many thousands of patients who would never have a problem would undergo treatment (with its attendant risks) but without any potential gain.

Certainly patients who have had a previous subarachnoid hemorrhage should undergo periodic screening because these patients have a higher risk of rupture of subsequent aneurysms that are found. Another easy decision would be an identical twin whose twin had a hemorrhage.

What about other situations that involve family members of patients who have had a subarachnoid hemorrhage? Experts do not recommend screening in patients who have just a single, first-degree relative with a subarachnoid hemorrhage. However, in patients who have had two or more relatives with a hemorrhage, the risk is higher; there is some genetic factor at play that makes aneurysms in this situation more likely to rupture. Here experts do recommend screening. Another situation in which screening is recommended is in patients with a kidney disorder called polycystic kidney disease.

The other factor that has to be considered is the psychological effects on a patient. Patients who think they have an aneurysm or know they have one (if they have undergone screening) may feel an overwhelming sense of anxiety. Some feel that they have a "time bomb" that could explode at any moment in their head. This is especially true if they have a relative who has already had a hemorrhage. In this situation, the patient should be referred to an expert in the field so that they can make the most informed decision possible.

For situations when screening is recommended, experts recommend using CTA or MRA. The accuracy of these tests, which are non-invasive, is approaching the accuracy of the full catheter angiogram. Nevertheless, because they are non-invasive, they have a much higher safety profile. However, after the test is done, if the angiogram does not show any aneurysms, doctors will often suggest repeating the test in five years to see if any abnormalities have developed. But what about if an aneurysm is found?

The AHA recommendations suggest that any symptomatic aneurysm should be considered for treatment. For small aneurysms in patients who have not had a previous subarachnoid hemorrhage, they recommend observation with follow-up angiograms to make sure the aneurysm is stable in size and shape. The size cutoff in the previously mentioned AHA guidelines is 10 mm, but some specialists would use the more conservative 7 mm cutoff. The guidelines suggest treatment for larger aneurysms and also for those aneurysms whose shape is worrisome. The most common worrisome shape is an aneurysm with a "daughter" sac, which means another, second area of outpouching that comes off the major aneurysm. These malformations are associated with a higher rupture rate.

As mentioned above, age and health of the patient are important factors to consider in deciding to fix the aneurysm or not.

PREVENTION OF HEMORRHAGIC STROKE

For hemorrhagic strokes, fewer preventative strategies exist. Preventing hypertensive intracranial bleeding, hemorrhagic stroke, involves the aggressive control of high blood pressure. The specific strategies are the same that were discussed above for ischemic stroke. This point should not be underestimated, but we will not repeat all of the information presented above. At present, there is no preventative therapy for patients with amyloid angiopathy.

However, for the ever-increasing anticoagulation-associated hemorrhages, very careful monitoring and control of the level of anticoagulation can prevent bleeding complications, including hemorrhagic stroke. It is well known that the higher the INR in patients on Coumadin, the higher the likelihood of bleeding. That is why the guidelines call for a very narrow range of the INR to be maintained. Strict maintenance of this narrow range is critical.

Years ago, when a patient took Coumadin, the individual doctor would get the result from the lab, and, if the INR was too high, he would order a reduction in the dose of Coumadin based on clinical judgment. Similarly, if the INR was too low, he would order an increase in the dose. There are problems with this system. Patients must keep their appointments and the lab must get the result to the doctor's office. Somebody in the office must get the information to the patient's chart and the doctor has to read it and then arrange for the patient to be notified about any changes in dosage. Most of the time this system, cumbersome as it is, works fine, but as you can imagine, there are many ways in which it could break down.

More recently, doctors and hospitals use "anticoagulation clinics," which are often run by nurses or pharmacists. These clinics take over the function of monitoring and dosing the Coumadin.

Some centers use computer algorithms to suggest dosing changes based on the last INR of the patient. Another strategy is to have patients measure their own INR at home using a home testing device. They can then report in by telephone to the central anticoagulation clinic, and most changes in dosage can be made over the phone. This strategy is especially useful in rural areas. Doctors have also come to better understand factors that change a patient's INR, such as dietary factors and other medicines that the patient may be taking. All of these steps have led to better anticoagulation control, which is important to both prevent hemorrhage and prevent the clotting problem for which the patient is using the Coumadin.

As for intracranial hemorrhage caused by discrete vascular lesions, we have already discussed preventing subarachnoid hemorrhage. For AVMs, treating these in any of the ways discussed in Chapter 7 will reduce the likelihood of subsequent bleeding. Regarding patients with CVST, primary prevention could become an issue if an incidental clot were found on a brain imaging study. In that case, anticoagulation would likely prevent a hemorrhagic stroke from occurring. In patients who have already presented with a clot or those who present with an arterial dissection, using heparin seems to work for secondary stroke prevention. The AHA guideline for arterial dissections is three to six months of anticoagulation therapy, followed by anti-platelet agents. Surgical repair or endovascular stenting of the injured vessel is sometimes required.

The reader can see that there are many ways to prevent strokes. This chapter is a long one, but its size reflects the importance of stroke prevention.

10

TIA: A Golden Opportunity at Stroke Prevention

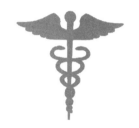

A s seen in the last chapter, the ability to actually prevent a stroke is an opportunity to save a person and their family from a potentially devastating ordeal that has lifelong consequences. Any opportunity to prevent a stroke from happening is a golden one.

Recall from Chapter 1 that a distinction was made between TIA and stroke in terms of the duration of symptoms. The TIA is defined just like a stroke except that all symptoms must resolve within twenty-four hours. So it is an abrupt onset of focal neurological symptoms that lasts less than twenty-four hours and that is caused by brain ischemia. But where does that twenty-four hour rule come from? And why is it twenty-four hours and not, say, twelve or forty-eight?

In the 1970s, the NIH sponsored a consensus conference to better define stroke and TIA. They drew together a prestigious group of neurologists, neurosurgeons, and neuropathologists. Their goal, with respect to TIA, was to create a working definition that would distinguish a transient episode of brain ischemia from permanent infarction. Specifically, they sought to distinguish two situations. The first is a temporary period of time when a portion of brain is not getting enough blood flow so that it is not working properly. The second is an area of brain that has been deprived of blood flow for long enough so that it dies and is not working. In the area of brain affected by a TIA, the notion was that, when blood flow was restored (naturally in this case), the function of that area of brain would normalize.

So with that goal clearly in mind, distinguishing temporary brain ischemia from permanent brain infarction, the group tried to decide on a time period. Because it was a definition, they had to choose some specific time threshold. As far back as the 1950s and 1960s, practicing neurologists knew for sure that the vast majority of TIA patients only had symptoms for less than one hour, often just ten to fifteen minutes in fact. However, they chose the twenty-four hour rule because they sought to distinguish transient ischemia from permanent infarction. At the time, this distinction made perfect sense because it did not affect treatments and we had no imaging techniques to show infarction.

However, over the past decade, three things have changed that have impacted this traditional definition of a TIA and, to a large extent, rendered it completely useless. The reader already knows about one of them: tPA. Because the time window for giving tPA is only three hours as of 2007, waiting for twenty-four hours to see whether someone has a TIA (rather than a stroke) makes absolutely no sense. Doctors must use tPA very rapidly for it to work.

The second thing that has changed from the 1970s is the advent of MRI to examine the brain in an entirely new way. The MRI shows the anatomy of the brain to a level of detail unimaginable twenty years ago. The MRI has the ability to distinguish transient ischemia from true permanent infarction, and by using MRI, doctors are finding that there actually is infarction that can occur much sooner than twenty-four hours. In fact, when an MRI is performed on TIA patients, doctors find that nearly half of them who meet the traditional definition for TIA have actually had a stroke. It is important to note that these are very small strokes and the patient will feel normal, but death (infarction) of brain cells has occurred. This finding has been shown in a half dozen different investigations.

Last, a study was published in 2000 suggesting that TIA patients have a high incidence of stroke in the short term. For decades, even in the 1970s, it was known that about 30 percent of TIA patients would suffer from a stroke in the next three to five years, but the 2000 study showed an unexpected finding. After a TIA, 10 percent of patients have strokes in the next ninety days, and half of those (5 percent of all TIA patients) have strokes within two days of their TIA. Numerous follow-up studies by other groups have verified this finding.

These three advancements—tPA treatment for stroke that must be given within three hours, knowing that a large proportion of TIAs are actually strokes according to MRI, and knowing that 5 percent of TIA patients will have a stroke within forty-eight hours—all changed the way that doctors view TIA. Together, all of these three advancements mean that using an arbitrary time (twenty-four hours) to distinguish between TIA and stroke is simply wrong.

Because of this, neurologists over the past several years have begun to suggest that the traditional definition of TIA be changed to "an episode of focal brain or retinal ischemia, usually lasting less than 1 hour, and in which there is no evidence of a stroke." This last part of the definition, no evidence of a stroke, implies that an imaging test such as CT or MRI has been done. It would classify some patients who have had (by the old definition) a TIA into a patient who has had (by the new definition) a stroke. It is important for the reader to know that, as of today, the traditional definition is still the one that is officially "on the books," but the reasons that are driving the new definition have changed the way doctors approach these patients.

Before the past several years, and to some extent even now, both patients and doctors have diminished the importance of a TIA. Terms such as "mini-stroke" and "transient" have led to minimizing the event. As a result, some patients do not seek medical care and, when they do, often very little is done about it. Surveys show that many people simply do not know what a TIA is and do not understand the significance of a TIA and what it may lead to.

This is all changing very rapidly.

Because the short-term risk of stroke after TIA is as high as 5–7 percent in the next forty-eight hours, doctors have begun to think of TIA patients much more as a medical emergency. This is important because, if one is going to prevent a stroke in a TIA patient, one must act rapidly.

One important part of the equation is better public education about just what a stroke is and what a TIA is. Increasingly, national societies such as the AHA and the National Stroke Association are spending more time, money, and effort in educating the American public about just what the signs of stroke and TIA are. They are also trying to get the word out that, if someone is having a TIA, they must immediately seek medical care. In addition, doctors have been working at more rapid evaluation.

Before doctors can evaluate patients with TIA, they have to diagnose them correctly. Furthermore, because most patients with TIA arrive at the ED or their doctors' offices completely asymptomatic, it is the history that doctors must focus on to make the diagnosis. The types of symptoms are exactly the same as the symptoms of stroke that we discussed in Chapter 3, but they most always last less than an hour. Doctors must try to distinguish these transient neurological symptoms from others that could mimic a TIA. These situations are the also the same as those that mimic stroke, also discussed in Chapter 3. Diagnosing TIA shows just how important taking a careful history is, because the physical examination will be normal and many of the usual tests will also be normal in the majority of TIA patients.

Once TIA is diagnosed, the doctor must decide what the cause is because the treatment depends on the underlying cause. Some TIAs are caused by blockage of the carotid artery in the neck (or less commonly, the vertebral artery). Some are caused by atrial fibrillation, and still others are associated with clots that go through an open foramen ovale in the heart. If this list sounds exactly like the causes of stroke, it is. This reinforces the concept that stroke and TIA are really different parts in the spectrum of the same disease.

However, on other occasions, despite a careful search, no cause is found. This is another similarity with stroke. Despite an exhaustive search, doctors do not find the cause in a substantial number of patients who have strokes.

That said, the careful search must be done, so it follows that TIA patients need to have several tests. These include some form of brain imaging (either a CT or an MRI), an ECG, a heart echo, and some test of their carotid arteries. Some hospitals will perform an ultrasound of the carotids to look for blockages. Others will do an angiogram using CT or MR. Each of these studies has advantages and disadvantages, but the important thing is to find out whether there is a high grade blockage.

Over the past decade, only a small percentage of TIA patients were admitted to the hospital for additional testing and treatments. In the 2000 study that was mentioned above, only 14 percent of patients were admitted! In another survey of ED visits for TIA across the whole country, researchers found that only 50 percent of patients with TIA were admitted. No study has found a higher number. In part, this relates to the fact that the perception is, all the patient is going to have done is to get an aspirin so why bother to hospitalize them? How will hospitalization help at all?

A lot of research has been done to try to risk-stratify patients with TIA, to try to understand which patients have a particularly elevated short-term risk, and which have a low risk. If such a system could be developed, then doctors could put the high-intensity resources such as hospitalization toward the patients with the highest risk and avoid it in those with especially low risk. Two different groups of researchers, one in California and another in England, have developed such grading systems over the past several years. The two systems were similar but not exactly the same. They found that some of the risk factors were older age, presence of diabetes and hypertension, and a longer duration of the TIA as well as symptoms that suggested that the cerebral hemispheres were affected.

Over time, these two groups of researchers collaborated to develop and test the so-called "ABCD^2" rule. Table 10.1 illustrates that rule. It is a seven-point

Table 10.1.
ABCD² Rule for Risk Stratification in TIA

Feature		Variable	Score
A	Age	≥60 years	1 point
B	Blood pressure	≥140/90	1 point
C	Clinical features	One-sided weakness	2 points
		Speech impairment and no weakness	1 point
D	Duration of TIA	≥60 minutes	2 points
		10–59 minutes	1 point
D	Diabetes	Present	1 point

scale that does a pretty good job of distinguishing low-risk from medium- and high-risk patients (see Table 10.2). Remarkably, 8 percent of patients with a high score, defined as 6–7 points, have a stroke within forty-eight hours of the TIA, and a total of 12 percent will have a stroke within a week. This rule is also very easy to use and remember.

Some physicians now admit all TIA patients to the hospital, but many others believe that only high-risk patients should be admitted. They think that the risk of stroke is low enough so that admitting all patients simply does not make economic sense. Over time, this practice is becoming less and less common, but, as of today, it still occurs at least 50 percent of the time. Going forward, it is very likely that physicians will use the ABCD² rule to decide which TIA patients need admission and which can be rapidly evaluated as outpatients.

The theory has been that, if TIA patients are admitted and rapidly evaluated for the various root causes, doctors can institute treatment for the underlying problem rapidly and thus prevent strokes. This is logical given what we now know about the short-term stroke risk. But is it true? Will admitting TIA patients accomplish this goal?

In October 2007, two studies were published that suggest that admitting patients for rapid diagnostic evaluation (and treatment) does lower the stroke

Table 10.2.
ABCD² Rule: What the Score Means

Risk level (points)	Percentage of patients	Risk of stroke at 2 days	Risk of stroke at 7 days
High (6–7)	21%	8%	12%
Moderate (4–5)	45%	4%	6%
Low (0–3)	34%	1%	1%

risk, by a very large amount. An English study of more than 1,200 patients tested the hypothesis that admitting TIA patients to the hospital would reduce the risk of stroke. All the patients admitted underwent a rapid evaluation and had treatments started if any specific cause was found. The ninety-day stroke rate fell from 10 percent to 2 percent, an 80 percent reduction in risk! Such a response is almost too good to be true, but the study was very well done and published in the prestigious journal *Lancet*.

That same month, another French study was also published that tested the same hypothesis and came up with the same results. More than 700 TIA patients were admitted to a rapid diagnostic evaluation unit, and if a treatable cause was found, that treatment was started as quickly as possible, often the same day. Using the $ABCD^2$ risk assessment tool, the patients in this study would have been expected to have a 6 percent risk of stroke. However, the actual ninety-day rate of stroke was just over 1 percent. The reduction in actual number of strokes was of the same order of magnitude as the British study.

What treatments should be administered?

All TIA patients should receive anti-platelet medication. The most commonly used one is something that is quite familiar: aspirin. Numerous studies have shown that aspirin reduces the rate of stroke in TIA patients by about 20–25 percent. Because it is very inexpensive and is effective in a very low dose (even one baby aspirin per day), which is unlikely to cause side effects, aspirin is often the doctors' first choice. We have seen that aspirin is also used in stroke patients, showing yet again the relationship of these two entities. Low doses work just as well as higher doses and have fewer side effects.

For all these reasons, aspirin is usually the first-line drug for TIA patients. However, some patients have allergies to aspirin, and others may get side effects even to the low dose used. In these situations, what are the other options? Clopidogrel is one. Doctors have had a lot of success with clopidogrel in cardiac patients. It is more expensive than aspirin, but the AHA recommends it as an alternative to aspirin. Logically, one might think the combination of clopidogrel and aspirin would work even better than either drug alone. Doctors tested this in a large study, but they were surprised by the results. They found a decrease in ischemic strokes, but they also found a corresponding increase in hemorrhagic strokes that more than overcame the reduction in ischemic events. At the present time, this combination is not recommended for TIA patients.

One combination that does work is aspirin plus a medicine called dipyridamole. This combination reduces stroke risk by another 20–25 percent compared with aspirin alone, and many doctors are using it preferentially to solely aspirin because of this additional benefit. That said, it does have more side effects and costs more than plain aspirin. Another drug called ticlodipine has been used but has fallen out of favor because of a poor side-effect profile. There are still many studies that are currently in progress to see whether other options or combinations are better than what is currently available.

As discussed in the last chapter, treating TIA patients with statin drugs most likely reduces stroke risk in TIA patients.

For TIA patients with atrial fibrillation, blood thinners are used to reduce the incidence of stroke. When the diagnosis is first made, patients usually receive intravenous heparin and are then switched over to oral Coumadin. The target INR is the same as that used for ischemic stroke: an INR of 2–3. For patients who cannot tolerate Coumadin, aspirin would be prescribed, and, as for stroke, TIA patients with the other causes of cardio-embolism (such as valvular disease or cardiomyopathy) would be similarly treated.

In some TIA patients with a PFO, aspirin is usually prescribed, but in some high-risk patients, if the aspirin is not working, full anticoagulation is used. Closing the opening between the two upper chambers of the heart (closing the PFO), either surgically or by one of the endovascular closure devices described in Chapter 9, is sometimes recommended, but the data that underlie this recommendation are weak. TIA from an arterial dissection is rare, and such patients would be treated the same as those with arterial dissection who have had a stroke.

The most important difference in the management of TIA patients, as opposed to those with stroke, is in those who have carotid stenosis. In TIA patients, operating to open the carotid or sometimes placing a stent to open the artery is important treatment. Because carotid surgery has been around for a few decades, there is much more information and experience with it. Stenting is a relatively new practice. The operation is called carotid endarterectomy, literally, removing the inside of the artery.

In this procedure, the surgeon makes an incision in the neck over the artery. He then cuts down to expose the carotid. After getting control of the blood vessel, he will open it up and remove the plaque that is causing the obstruction. Last, he sews the artery closed and closes the skin incision. After the procedure, the patient is given blood thinners to keep the operated blood vessel open. As you might imagine, there are risks of this surgery, especially because it is generally done on elderly people who have other medical problems. A very small percentage of patients die from the surgery, and several percent will have a stroke that is a direct complication of the procedure.

This operation has been shown to reduce the incidence of stroke considerably in patients who have very-high-grade blockages. Several very large studies done in the late 1980s and 1990s showed that performing carotid endarterectomy in patients with carotid blockages more than 70 percent reduced the risk of stroke by a very large amount. The absolute risk reduction was 17 percent, meaning that of one hundred patients with blockages, seventeen fewer patients who had the operation would have a stroke compared with those who were treated with the best medical management. This degree of treatment effect is quite large; many major changes in practice that doctors have instituted have been made for absolute improvements of 1–2 percent.

For this treatment effect to work, the downside risk of the surgery itself must be low. The major risks of the surgery are death, stroke, and injury to some important nerves in the neck. Therefore, carotid endarterectomy must be done by experienced vascular surgeons who have a low complications rate. What about endovascular stenting? In this procedure, a physician with specialized training inserts a catheter into the groin and threads it to the carotid artery in the neck. When he is inside the vessel at the point of the stenosis, or blockage, he deploys the stent.

Intuitively, it would seem that the complication rate would be lower if open surgery, as opposed to stenting, could be avoided, but so far, the results are mixed. One major study showed that the outcomes with stenting were actually worse than those with endarterectomy. Most of the other studies showed equivalent results, but because the open surgical approach has been the standard treatment for two decades, many favor this approach. The one measure that consistently gets better results with stenting is cranial nerve damage. It is logical that endovascular stenting would create less injury to nerves coursing through the neck than open surgery. Studies are still ongoing to clarify which procedure is best for which patients.

These studies will focus on which device ought to be used (there are several), how much training is required before doctors can safely perform the procedure (technique is very important), and who the best target patient population is (everyone or just patients with high surgical risk).

Whichever procedure the patient undergoes, it is clear that sooner is better. In the past, doctors would often wait weeks to months to perform the carotid surgery, but newer data that we have discussed above make it clear that earlier surgery is better with respect to stroke prevention. Once again, this is consistent with the paradigm shift for faster stroke care in general.

11

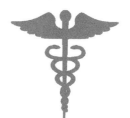

New Horizons: Bats and Snakes

As with nearly every subject in medicine, there is a continual search for newer and better ways of diagnosing and treating patients. Physicians from across the globe are actively seeking novel ways to care for stroke patients. The amount of research reports that are published every month is staggering.

For ischemic stroke, this research is driven, in part, by the fact that only a very small number of patients are treated with tPA. There are several reasons for this, the main two being the narrow time window (three hours) as well as the doctors' fear about bleeding complications. Therefore, researchers are trying to find strategies that address both of these issues; they are looking for treatments that can be given beyond the three-hour window and that are safer with respect to hemorrhage rate. Another issue with these new horizons in therapy is the fact that, even if tPA is successful at opening up the blocked artery, the artery can form clot again. Therefore, not only is it important to get the artery open but to keep it open.

In this chapter, we will touch on a few of the areas that appear most promising and most interesting, and we will break these new horizons into three categories: new care delivery systems, new medical approaches, and new interventional or surgical approaches. Doctors are combining some of these approaches, and we will discuss that aspect as well.

STROKE SYSTEMS OF CARE

We reviewed the concept of stroke centers in a previous chapter, but it is important to recognize that not every hospital can be a stroke center, although smaller hospitals can safely administer tPA. However, there are not enough neurologists across the country who have expertise in acute stroke care to supply neurological consultation for all the patients who present themselves to smaller, perhaps more rural, EDs.

One advancement that is being used to a small extent now but will likely be used to an even greater extent in the future is telemedicine. Using broadband cable to connect smaller hospitals with larger more centralized ones, the specialists in the large comprehensive stroke centers can supply real-time consultation to emergency physicians and internists seeing acute stroke patients. Using equipment similar to a webcam, specialists from the big city can "virtually" examine a patient hundreds of miles away and actually do an NIH stroke scale on them. The neurologist can have the digitized CT scan sent over the same cables to look for hemorrhage.

Based on this information, the consulting neurologist can assist the on-site doctor to make a decision that the on-site physician might not have been comfortable making without this help. This telemedicine concept has been used in several areas in both the United States and abroad; the proof of concept has been demonstrated. Over time, it is very likely that this paradigm will be used in more locations.

NEW MEDICAL APPROACHES TO STROKE TREATMENT

Expanding the Indications for tPA in Ischemic Stroke

Currently, doctors who give tPA to patients with acute ischemic stroke do so only if they can treat the patient within three hours from the onset of symptoms, and this is how the FDA has licensed tPA in the United States. In addition, as it stands, the only imaging test that the emergency physician needs is a regular CT scan of the brain. The major purpose is to exclude a brain hemorrhage. However, the CT does not tell doctors how much brain tissue is at risk or whether the blood vessel is blocked or open. Over the past few years, doctors have been experimenting with other ways of safely expanding this narrow three-hour time window, yet another variable that is being investigated is the length of the tPA intravenous infusion. Presently, the full dose is given over sixty minutes, but some data suggest that giving the same dose over a ninety-minute period may lead to improved results.

At this time, there are two studies that are looking at using tPA in the customary dose but beyond three hours from onset of symptoms. The reason for this is that reanalysis of some of the original studies that we discussed in Chapter 6 suggested a possible benefit beyond three hours. An ECASS 3 study is looking at tPA treatment from three to four and a half hours after onset, and the Third International Stroke Trial is a randomized trial of patients being treated with standard tPA up to six hours out from the onset of symptoms. These studies have been carefully designed in terms of the number of subjects enrolled so that they will be able to answer the important question of how long the time window should be for tPA therapy.

Another way that stroke specialists are trying to extend the time window is by using advanced imaging studies such as MRA and CTA. The purpose of these tests is not primarily to exclude a bleed but to better define exactly what is going on in an individual patient. How much brain tissue is already dead? Is the responsible artery open or blocked? How much brain tissue is currently ischemic (not getting enough blood flow) but not yet infarcted; that is to say, how much tissue is at risk? MRI can tell doctors this information.

The MRI will indicate what doctors call the ischemic penumbra (see Figure 11.1). This concept is important to understand. When a stroke occurs, there is a central area of dead, infarcted tissue that at the present time is not salvageable. Surrounding this area is a region of brain that is salvageable. It is this tissue that doctors focus on; they try to minimize or, if possible, eliminate this ischemic penumbra. The MRI defines the central infarction and the surrounding ischemic area, and the theory is that treatment for some patients with a favorable MRI profile, even after three hours, is safe and effective if used in the right circumstances.

For example, if the artery is blocked and there is a large amount of brain tissue at risk, a patient may benefit from tPA use at four or five hours or possibly even longer after onset. Conversely, some MRA and CTA may identify those whose arteries have already opened up spontaneously. In this group of patients, there is no need to give tPA because its only purpose is to open the vessel, so why take the risk from tPA when there is no chance of benefit? Another fairly common situation is when patients wake up with stroke symptoms. Because doctors do not know when the onset of symptoms was, they must assume that the "last time seen normal" was the time of onset, making almost all these patients ineligible for tPA. MRA and CTA can also aid in identifying the status of these patients who might be treatable with tPA based on these advanced imaging studies.

Preliminary work suggests that this strategy may be quite useful in safely and effectively treating patients farther out from the onset of symptoms (or

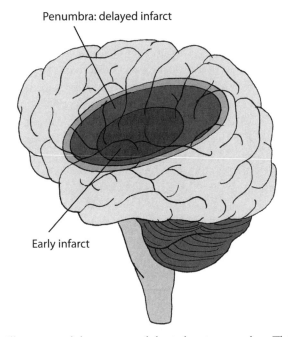

Penumbra: delayed infarct

Early infarct

Figure 11.1. Illustration of the concept of the ischemic penumbra. This penumbra is the area of tissue that is ischemic but not infarcted. It surrounds a central core of already infarcted tissue. It is the outer penumbra that is the target for tPA and other reperfusion therapies. When blood flow is restored, the ischemic penumbra is salvaged. Doctors are using MRI and CT perfusion studies to define the volume of the penumbra.

with an unclear time of onset) than the current FDA guidelines suggest. In one German study of 174 patients, all patients arriving within six hours of stroke onset had an MRI to see whether there was a large ischemic penumbra. Those who were treated using these MRI findings did better than the ones in which the standard CT was used. Two other trials are currently underway to further test this novel use of MRI to help extend the time window for tPA use.

New Thrombolytics Drugs

Teneteplase is a mutant form of tPA that lasts longer (has a longer half-life) in the body and seems to be more specific in its binding to fibrin. These two properties may make it a safer and more effective thrombolytic drug. An early phase 2 study had favorable results, and another randomized trial is currently underway.

Desmoteplase is made from the saliva of vampire bats. In a trial using MRI criteria (as above), desmoteplase was used for patients in the three to nine hour window after symptom onset. Although the first part of the study had high bleeding rates, the second part, when dosing was more carefully calculated, showed very favorable outcomes. However, the phase 3 study results were reported recently (although not published in a scientific journal yet) and showed disappointing results.

The researchers, a team from both the United States and Europe, found that the poor and unexpected results may result simply from the play of chance. The placebo group (no treatment) did exceptionally well in this study, which makes it more difficult to show an improvement with the experimental group who received the desmoteplase. As well, the deaths in the desmoteplase group were late and not associated with brain hemorrhages. Many of them were non-neurological deaths, suggesting that it was not the desmoteplase that contributed to them. Although desmoteplase is clearly not something that can be recommended outside of the study setting, the investigators are still trying to sort out the data to explain their findings.

Another new agent comes from the pit viper, one of the most venomous snakes known to man. Its venom is a fibrinolytic drug. That is how the snake kills its prey; its victim bleeds to death. Despite this, the drug, called ancrod, seems to have a reduced bleeding rate compared with tPA in experiments done on stroke patients. Preliminary studies of larger groups of patients treated up to six hours after symptom onset, however, have been disappointing.

Combinations of Medications

Another way that doctors have been trying to improve the results of tPA is by using the drug in combination with other anti-thrombotic drugs: anti-platelet agents and other anticoagulants. Because blood platelets help form blood clots, one strategy used is to combine tPA with various types of anti-platelet therapies. In these experiments, the anti-platelet drugs used are intravenous medicines that are much more powerful than those referred to in Chapter 10. They are a class of drug called glycoprotein IIb/IIIa inhibitors (referred to as 2B-3A inhibitors). Various preliminary work suggests that combining tPA and 2B-3A inhibitors is safe and may increase the rate at which the blocked artery stays open after treatment. One ongoing study is testing a 2B-3A inhibitor, combined with aspirin plus a form of heparin after tPA.

Yet another trial is studying tPA followed by argatroban, an anticoagulant that directly inhibits the formation of a clot. Very preliminary data in a small number of patients are promising and have showed an increased rate of unblocking the target artery. All of these combinations, although showing some potential, are still experimental and by no means part of standard care as of this time.

Neuroprotectants

We have seen in previous chapters the dismal track record of a large group of medications called neuroprotectants, drugs that protect brain cells from dying after an ischemic event. Some physicians feel that some of the older trials failed because of poor study designs, not necessarily because of a problem with the compounds being studied. So despite those grim results, there are ongoing studies of newer neuroprotectants. There are several target biochemical pathways that lead a neuron from ischemic insult to final death. They relate to the cell integrity of the neurons, the production of inflammatory chemicals, and oxygen free radicals. Each of these can contribute to cell death.

Recently, the antibiotic "minocycline" was reported to help stroke patients. Minocycline is a tetracycline-group antibiotic sometimes used for acne treatment. Why would this work in stroke? The proposed mechanism is not minocycline's antibiotic effect but other effects that are anti-inflammatory. It impacts the levels of a variety of mediators of cell death. Thus, its use is being studied as a neuroprotective agent.

A recent small Israeli study of 152 patients showed that giving oral minocycline within six to twenty-four hours after acute stroke improved the clinical outcomes of these patients. They measured better NIH stroke scores and modified Rankin scores in more patients who received minocycline than in placebo. The improvement was seen within a week of the event. Although these results were very robust and very promising, there have been many studies on neuroprotectants that looked good in animal studies or in preliminary human studies only to be proved ineffective in larger, scientifically rigorous studies. Obviously, more research needs to be done on larger numbers of patients to really know whether this therapy is of any real benefit or not.

Another focus of study involves using "caffeinol": a combination of caffeine and alcohol. This unlikely combination produced some impressive effects on rats. Human studies are ongoing. Various anti-inflammatory drugs are being tested as well. Many, including steroids, have been shown to be without value, but other anti-inflammatory drugs continue to be studied. Much of the early results in this particular area have not produced any striking information, but other experiments are still ongoing, including one with interferon, a substance that is already approved for use in patients with multiple sclerosis.

Albumin, a protein that is a normal component of our blood, is being tested because it inhibits oxygen free-radical production and also may help with blood flow through the microcirculation of the brain. There is also some suggestion that there is synergism between tPA and albumin. Another drug, glyceryl trinitrate, is being tested because of its favorable effect on nitric acid levels and ability to improve perfusion in the ischemic penumbra.

Other drugs currently being tested are piclozotan (a serotonin receptor antagonist similar to medicines used for migraine headache), magnesium (which has failed in other trials but is now being tested very early, even being given by paramedics in ambulances), and citicoline (a drug aimed at stabilizing the cell membranes of neurons and their supporting cells). Yet another drug is Lovastatin, which falls into the category of drugs called statins that we learned about in the chapter on prevention. This medication is being tested not because of its effects on cholesterol but because it also increases nitric oxide levels and, like minocycline, has some anti-inflammatory activity. Additionally, the whole group of statin drugs seem to improve endothelial cell function (the cells that line blood vessels) and also improve blood flow. You can expect additional trials of this important group of drugs, especially because they are already FDA approved for other indications.

Induced hypothermia (which we will discuss later in this chapter) is also being tested in combination with tPA. Another treatment, discussed in Chapter 5, blood sugar control, is also being tested in a more rigorous study looking at the benefit of very tight control of blood sugar levels.

Gene Therapy

Gene therapy is a promising strategy for cerebrovascular diseases. Ultimately, the events that occur in the brain (as in the rest of the body) occur at a cellular level. Cell ischemia, infarction, the process of atherosclerotic plaque formation, as well as the development of cerebral aneurysms are all cellular processes. Biochemical events occur; proteins are synthesized and degraded. At the heart of all these processes, many of which are poorly understood, are genes. Genes are bits of DNA that code for the synthesis of individual proteins. These genes code for proteins that mediate neuroprotection of brain cells, inhibition of thrombosis, and stimulation of new blood vessel growth after an ischemic event.

Scientists are beginning to understand how to deliver synthesized genes into patients so that newer, healthier response proteins can be manufactured rather than the older, unhealthy ones. Gene therapy is truly at the forefront of modern biology and is a hot topic, because it is being used for many different diseases such as heart attack, degenerative diseases such as Parkinson's syndrome, and others.

In subarachnoid hemorrhage, investigators are also experimenting with gene therapy to try to improve the results of endovascular therapy by modulating the underlying biology that leads to thrombosis of the clot in the coiled aneurysm. In other experiments, genes that affect vascular nitric oxide levels have been manipulated to improve the healing that occurs after injury to the inner layer of arteries.

Gene therapy is still in its infancy, and there are numerous problems still to work out with it before it is ready for routine patient use. Of course with any promising therapy that is long range, there is the possibility that it will never be useful. However, if the bugs are worked out, gene therapy is a potential way of truly fixing the underlying biological problems as opposed to simply fixing the gross manifestations of stroke.

Hypothermia

Perhaps you have heard stories about people who have fallen into a freezing cold lake in winter and, despite being under water for long periods of time, they survive, often neurologically intact. Or consider how a hibernating bear's brain is protected during the winter despite the bear's heartbeat and blood pressure dipping down to levels that could kill the animal if it was active. Doctors have long known that hypothermia can protect the brain while fever, conversely, at least in stroke patients, leads to worse outcomes.

Normal body temperature is between 36 and 37 degrees centigrade. Mild (34–36 degrees centigrade) and moderate (32–34 degrees centigrade) hypothermia not only decrease the demand for oxygen but also have other beneficial effects. These include some neuroprotectant effects as well as reducing damage caused by oxygen free radicals. Several large studies have shown that induced hypothermia in comatose survivors of cardiac arrest improves mortality rates and neurological outcomes.

Although no studies in acute ischemic stroke have shown a clear-cut benefit of inducing hypothermia in humans, in animals hypothermia has been shown to reduce the volume of infarcted tissue. Newer methods of inducing hypothermia are being studied as are various methods of preventing some of its adverse effects, most notably shivering and infection.

The main two ways to cool a patient are with external cooling and by internal cooling.

In the former, there is a product called the "Arctic Sun," which has pads placed on the patient's body. Cool water is pumped through the pads, and this leads to a lowered body temperature. The advantage of this technique is that it is quick and does not rely on very high-tech maneuvers. However, it is uncomfortable for the patient and requires sedation, which interferes with the neurological evaluation.

The second type of device is endovascular, in which a special catheter is inserted into the large femoral vein in the groin. This catheter contains a cooling tube that lowers the body temperature. The advantage of this technique is that it allows the doctor to precisely control the patient's temperature, but the disadvantage is that this large catheter is an invasive procedure. There have been some studies of hypothermia in other types of brain injury (such as post-cardiac arrest and traumatic brain injury). One study in patients with subarachnoid hemorrhage did not show benefit of hypothermia, but more work is being done for ischemic stroke.

Other investigational treatments for ischemic stroke include photo-therapy, in which near-infrared light energy is applied to the head. These photons penetrate several centimeters below the skin and skull and are thought to have an impact on physiological processes. There have been some promising findings in animal experiments.

Another strategy is called "cortical stimulation." This relates to the concept of "neuroplasticity." The old electrical (neuronal) circuits that are damaged are rerouted to other areas of normally functioning brain. This rerouting can be augmented by repetitive movement and practice such as that gained from physical therapy, but it can also be accomplished by the application of an electrical current. One experimental cortical stimulation device that is being tested is something like a cardiac pacemaker. A battery pack and pulse generator are implanted in the chest wall, and the active lead is put on the outer surface of the dura. Low-level electrical stimulation is delivered. Like with many of these experimental therapies, there is some initial promising data, but it is entirely too early to draw any firm conclusions. Some physicians are even testing the effects of magnetic fields applied to the head to see whether there is any cortical stimulation from that, again with some early evidence of benefit. Yet another group is looking at using a robotic device that simulates the effects of physical therapy.

Another technique that scientists have studied is increasing the amount of oxygen delivered to the ischemic brain. One method that has been studied over the past two decades is the delivery of hyperbaric oxygen, which is oxygen at higher than atmospheric pressures. The patient is placed in a pressurized chamber to increase the ambient pressure and increase oxygen delivery. Despite decades of investigation, the role of hyperbaric oxygen is still unclear, in both stroke and many other medical conditions. Although this is just oxygen, there is still toxicity involved with these high levels of oxygen.

NEW SURGICAL AND INTERVENTIONAL ENDOVASCULAR APPROACHES

Endovascular Therapies

The current paradigm for treating heart attacks is to open the blocked artery as rapidly as possible. The preferred method is to take the patient to the cardiac catheterization lab and thread a tiny catheter into the coronary artery, break up the clot, and then stent the blocked area. When these facilities are not available, intravenous tPA is used. Currently with stroke, the paradigm is the opposite; use tPA first and, if the patient presents beyond three hours after symptom onset or has a contra-indication, use intra-arterial tPA. In part, this is because there are far fewer physicians trained to do brain catheterization compared with those who can do heart catheterization. It is also because of the fact that the quality and quantity of the scientific studies in stroke patients do not compare with those done in cardiac patients.

Several studies have examined using intra-arterial tPA, but this is not yet an FDA-approved strategy. In this treatment, the doctor will insert a catheter into the femoral artery in the groin and feed it all the way into the brain. Once there, a variety of things can be accomplished. First, the status of the brain-feeding arteries can be assessed by performing an angiogram. Second, if there is a blockage, tPA can be administered locally to the clot in smaller doses than would be used intravenously.

Third, a stent can be deployed (just as in cardiac interventions; see Figure 11.2). Last, various devices can be used to physically remove the clot. One such device, called the MERCI clot retriever, is already FDA approved. It looks like a tiny corkscrew at the end of the catheter. The corkscrew is

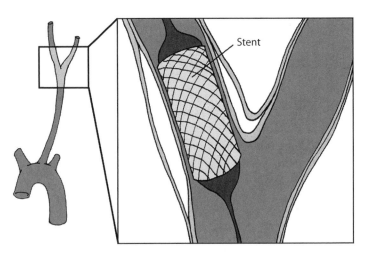

Figure 11.2. Illustration of how a carotid stent is deployed. The dark gray shows a balloon on a catheter that will be blown up to expand the atherosclerotic lesion. Next, the mesh-like stent is expanded so that it maintains the carotid artery open. Carotid stenting of blocked carotids is becoming more commonly used, but surgical carotid endarterectomy is still the standard therapy.

advanced into the clot and then it is withdrawn. When it works as designed, the clot backs out just as a cork backs out of a wine bottle. There are other devices that use suction, a mechanical snare, laser technology, and ultrasound energy to either break up the clot or remove it. In the case of ultrasound-tipped catheters, the energy is thought to loosen the fibrin strands in the clot and to exert a pressure between the catheter and the clot. Both of these improve the penetration of the locally delivered tPA into the offending clot.

Finally, there are combinations of therapy. Some doctors will give a smaller than normal dose of intravenous tPA and then take the patient to the catheterization lab to open up the clot with intra-arterial tPA, with or without one of the other devices described in the last paragraph. As well, once the clot is removed by any of these techniques, the artery itself can be opened by inflating a tiny balloon (angioplasty) and then deploying a rigid stent to keep the artery from closing off again.

We know that patients with atrial fibrillation form clot in their left atrium and that this clot can embolize to the brain and cause stroke. Traditional anticoagulation works fairly well, but this therapy has many side effects, the most worrisome being bleeding. Doctors are actively studying newer anticoagulants that are safer and easier to use. This group of medicines is called direct thrombin inhibitors. They are easier to use than Coumadin and are not affected by as many foods or other drugs. Early trials suggest they are at least as safe as Coumadin, although there is some concern about liver damage from the drugs. The one that is the most thoroughly tested is called ximelagatran.

In atrial fibrillation, most of the clot forms in a small appendage of the left atrium (the left atrial appendage), a region that is like an outpouching that creates sluggish flow. This creates another potential strategy. Doctors have invented various devices that can be inserted endovascularly, again through the groin, and that can then be deployed into the left atrial appendage where it remains, essentially obliterating the appendage so that there is no space for clot. The same goal can be accomplished surgically, but obviously if it can be done without open surgery, all the better.

Similar devices exist for patients with PFO. The common thread is that a catheter is inserted into the heart, and the opening between the right and left atria is crossed by the catheter. The device is then deployed, closing off the hole. There are studies today that are testing these devices. Until the results of these studies are released, we will not know which, if any, are superior to medical therapy or open surgical therapy.

Another novel device is a large catheter that contains two large balloons, which is placed into the aorta by way of the femoral artery. The balloons are partially inflated. This leads to an increase in blood flow toward the brain (and decreased flow in the legs). This increased flow is meant to overcome the diminished flow in the ischemic brain. The device is currently undergoing safety trials and has been shown to increase CBF by 30–40 percent.

In the field of treating carotid artery stenosis to prevent stroke in TIA patients, open surgical procedure remains the standard treatment. However, there is a continual flow of new medical devices being tested. We touched on this latter issue in Chapter 10 on TIA. New types of stents and newer devices to prevent small emboli from being released at the time of stenting (called embolic protection devices) are being studied. Hopefully, the results of a number of studies that are currently ongoing will settle some of these issues going forward.

Surgical Treatments

For patients with very large strokes, both ischemic and hemorrhagic, sometimes there is so much brain swelling that the patient dies from the effects of this increased pressure. In some settings, surgeons will do a heroic procedure called a decompressive hemicraniectomy (see Figure 11.3). The surgeon removes a piece of the skull (temporarily) to accommodate new swelling. In

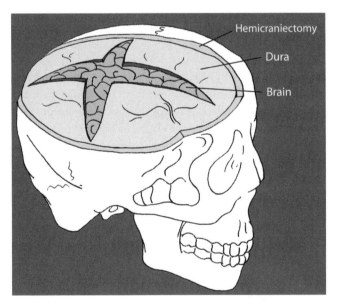

Figure 11.3. The radical surgical procedure of decompressive hemicraniectomy. This is used as a last-ditch effort to treat elevated intracranial pressure. The piece of skull that is removed is often implanted beneath the patient's skin to keep it alive and prevent it from becoming infected. The dura is opened so that the underlying brain swelling will not press against the dura or skull.

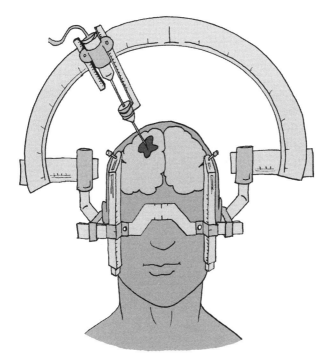

Figure 11.4. An intracranial hemorrhage (dark gray). The outer circular apparatus is used for positioning of the endoscopic instrument. The scope is then inserted into the hemorrhage, and the blood is aspirated using a syringe.

some patients who would otherwise die, this procedure may work. The piece of skull is later replaced in those patients who do survive. Results from clinical trials suggest that younger patients operated on early (before there is too much irreversible brain damage) may benefit from this procedure. These decisions must be made on a case-by-case basis.

When neurosurgeons do intervene, they are increasingly using less invasive techniques, the data from the last chapter notwithstanding. Like abdominal and chest surgeons, neurosurgeons are using endoscopic techniques (see Figure 11.4) to reduce the morbidity of surgery. One technique is used on patients who develop elevated ICP from hydrocephalus caused by blocked spinal fluid flow. Surgeons will occasionally use an endoscopic technique to relieve this pressure.

CONCLUSIONS

It is important to know that some of the medications and devices referred to in this chapter are entirely experimental and are not used in routine clinical practice. Many of them may fail in phase 3 clinical trials and never be used in clinical practice. Other devices that we have referred to are close to being ready for routine clinical use; others are not FDA approved but are being used in an "off-label" manner, which means that they are legal to use for one indication but doctors are using them for another.

The investigation of stroke is a continually evolving field. Over time, physicians and scientists will find better ways of treating strokes and, most importantly, of preventing them.

Timeline

The reason of an Apoplexy, and the cause of so sudden a Deprivation of Life, that great Judge, the Prince of Physicians, Hippocrates, resolves into a Stagnation or Station of the Blood, whereby all Motion and Action of the Spirits is taken away … and that its Motion is stop'd either by sharp Humours, or a Plethora, or an Afflux of cold Humours; the last of which he makes not so sudden.

> —attributed to B. Allen, 1699, showing how the Hippocratic notions of disease being caused by imbalance in the "humors" persisted well into the Middle Ages

5000 BC   The practice of drilling a hole in the skull, known as trephination, is used to release evil spirits, although it is unclear whether this procedure was used for stroke, but some evidence exists that cavemen did this for bad headache. This procedure is similar to what modern neurosurgeons do to treat some forms of hemorrhagic stroke.

1500 BC   The Ebers Papyrus, the most important of the ancient Egyptian medical papyri, describes some brain anatomy but says nothing of stroke. As a step in preparing mummies, the Egyptian embalmers would remove the entire brain through the nose. Of note, some surgeons now surgically remove the pituitary gland via the nose. As well, this shows the sophistication that the ancients had with respect to brain anatomy. On this subject, the Ebers scribe wrote,

> If thou examines a man having a gaping wound in his head penetrating to the bone, smashing his skull, and rending open the brain of his skull, thou shouldst palpate his wound. Shouldst thou find that smash which in his skull like those corrugations which form in molten copper, and something therein throbbing and fluttering under thy fingers, like the weak place of an infant's crown before it becomes whole—when it has happened there is no throbbing and fluttering under thy fingers until the brain of his skull is rent open and he discharges blood from both his nostrils, and he suffers with stiffness in his neck.

460 BC The great ancient Greek physician Hippocrates thinks all disease is related to an imbalance in the four "humors" of the body (phlegm, blood, black bile, and yellow bile). He believes the brain is responsible for intelligence and sensation. The Greeks use the word "apoplexy" to name stroke, a word suggesting that a force outside of the body is responsible.

280 BC Erasistratus, of Chios, Greece, describes the divisions of the brain.

160 AD Galen, another Greek physician who practiced in Rome, was probably the most well-known physician since Hippocrates. An empiric scientist, he dissected animals and described some of the large veins of the brain that are now known to be involved in cerebral venous sinus thrombosis. In 171 AD, he gives a lecture on the brain.

1536 Nicholo Massa studies the cerebrospinal fluid (that the Egyptians had described about three millennia before).

1543 Andreas Vesalius, a famous anatomist, describes the pineal gland and other brain structures.

1573 Constanzo Varolio names the pons, a part of the brainstem, and begins dissecting the brain from its base.

1658	Johann Jakob Wepfer, a Swiss physician, first suggests that stroke is caused by broken blood vessels in the brain. He was also the first to suggest that not enough blood from an arterial blockage could cause a stroke. His ideas came from postmortem studies.
1664	Thomas Willis, an English physician and anatomist, publishes his famous treatise on brain anatomy, *Cerebri Anatome*. He is the first to describe the circle of arteries at the base of the brain named after him.
1695	Humphrey Ridley publishes one of the first comprehensive studies of brain anatomy.
1732	N. Robinson recommends blood letting, a popular treatment for many maladies to treat stroke.
1820	J. Cooke continues to recommend blood letting, writing that, in these circumstances (speaking of stroke), "what practice could be more rational than abstracting [removing] blood speedily and freely?"
1823	Marie-Jean-Pierre Flourens first describes the role of the cerebellum.
1831	Richard Bright publishes an atlas of brain and nervous system disease that included data from more than 200 specimens that he had collected.
1895	Henrick Quincke first uses the lumbar puncture to study the cerebrospinal fluid and to diagnose brain diseases.
Late 1800s	Rudolph Virchow, a brilliant German pathologist, begins to sort out the importance of the arterial wall in cerebral thrombosis and embolism and clearly shows that arterial obstruction results in stroke.
Late 1800s to early 1900s	Canadian physician William Osler describes the pathological findings in all kinds of strokes, including endocarditis, a common cause of stroke during that era. He later goes on to be one of the founders of the Johns Hopkins University medical school. In 1892, Osler recommends blood letting as a method to reduce the blood pressure in cases of stroke. As well, Jules Dejerine and Charles Foix begin to study and describe the

relationship of specific brain lesions and specific clinical syndromes. This is called "clinico-pathological correlation."

1935   Osler's *Principles and Practice of Medicine* (a textbook started by Osler and taken over by many of his protégés after his death in 1919) finally and specifically states that blood letting is of no practical value in treating stroke.

1946   Drs. Raymond Adams and Charles Kubik describe basilar artery occlusion and the difference between thrombosis in a vessel and an embolism of clot that travels from one artery to another.

1970s to the present   Modern databases and stroke registries begin to flourish and help propel research into the current age, allowing doctors to learn more information about the way stoke presents and the risk factors for stroke.

1980s   Large studies show that surgical treatment to relieve a blockage in the carotid artery in the neck will decrease the chance of stroke.

1990   After enormous strides in understanding heart disease in the 1970s and 1980s, U.S. President George Bush pronounces the 1990s the "Decade of the Brain."

1995   The first positive study for a specific medication, the National Institute of Neurological Diseases and Stroke trial, showing that tissue plasminogen activator (tPA) works to improve the outcomes of patients with ischemic stroke, is published in the *New England Journal of Medicine*. Within a year, this becomes "standard of care" but is used very infrequently because of controversy about its safety.

2000   The first article to suggest that up to 5 percent of transient ischemic attack (TIA) patients will have a stroke within the next forty-eight hours is published. This is much higher than previously realized, and later studies confirm this finding. This stimulates research into stroke prevention by aggressive treatment of TIA patients.

2000 to the present   Multiple new therapies and medical devices are being tested. Brain aneurysms are being treated with endovascular coils (obviating the need for open surgery). Doctors test new procoagulant drugs to make the blood clot easier in cases of hemorrhagic stroke. Devices to keep arteries open, called "stents," frequently used in cardiac disease, are used in brain arteries. Brain catheterization to deliver tPA directly into or near the clot in the brain is studied and used clinically. Many other treatments are being tested as well.

Glossary

Words that appear in **boldface** in the definitions are also found in the glossary.

Aneurysm: An aneurysm is a weak spot, or an outpouching in an artery. These occur in arteries all over the body. They are like a weak spot in a tire that balloons out. Just as in a tire, if the pressure in an aneurysm gets too high, the aneurysm can rupture. In the case of cerebral aneurysms, the blood resulting from rupture leaks into the subarachnoid space and causes a subarachnoid hemorrhage.

Angiogram: An angiogram is an x-ray of a blood vessel, almost always an artery. Historically, an angiogram, sometimes called an arteriogram, was done by a specialist in radiology who would put a thin catheter into an artery and then thread it to the artery of interest. Once there, the radiologist injects a dye that will show up on the x-ray, which will give an actual picture of the artery itself. Increasingly, doctors are using **CT scan** and **MRI** to get pictures of the blood vessels.

Anterior circulation: The anterior circulation refers to the blood vessels in the front of the brain. This is mostly the portion of the brain fed by the two carotid arteries that arise in the neck and then enter the brain. These arteries and their branches feed the cerebrum and some other parts of the brain. The anterior circulation is connected to the **posterior circulation** by the **Circle of Willis**.

Anticoagulant: When you cut yourself, your blood will clot, or coagulate. Sometimes, clots can form inside a vein and travel from one part of the body to another; this situation is called an embolism and is a common cause of stroke. Anticoagulants are medications prescribed by doctors to make the blood thinner and less likely to clot. In certain situations, such as **atrial fibrillation**, anticoagulants can prevent strokes.

Anti-platelet medications: Platelets are components of blood that help it to clot or coagulate. Anti-platelet medications make platelets less sticky and help to prevent clots. You are all familiar with at least one anti-platelet drug: aspirin. There are others such as clopidogrel and dipyridamole. These medications are used for stroke (as well as heart attack) prevention.

Aorta: The aorta is the major artery of the body that arises from the heart and is the origin of the two **carotid arteries** and the two **vertebral arteries**.

Aphasia: Aphasia is the loss of the ability to understand language or to speak. In stroke, this is caused by **infarction** of the portion of the brain that serves as the speech centers.

Arachnoid membrane: The arachnoid membrane is the middle of the three membranes that make up the **meninges**. Just beneath this layer is the subarachnoid space where the **cerebrospinal fluid** lies.

Arterial dissection: Arteries have three layers. Sometimes, blood will split the three layers. This is called an arterial dissection and can lead to either rupture of the blood vessel (causing **hemorrhagic stroke**) or clotting within the blood vessel (causing **ischemic stroke**).

Arteriovenous malformation (AVM): An AVM is an abnormal tangle of blood vessels whereby there is an abnormal connection between an artery and a vein. These can occur anywhere in the body. In the brain, they can lead to stroke (usually hemorrhagic) and seizures.

Atherosclerosis: Atherosclerosis is the pathological process in the body whereby plaques containing cholesterol and other blood components form in arteries. This leads to partial or complete blockages in the arteries, which decreases the flow of blood distally. In the brain, this can lead to an **ischemic stroke**.

Atrial fibrillation: Atrial fibrillation is a chaotic rhythm of the top chambers of the heart called the atria. Because the atria lose the ability to pump in a coordinated manner, clots form. Because these clots can become loose and travel to the brain (**embolism**), atrial fibrillation is a very important risk factor for **ischemic stroke**.

Autoregulation: Autoregulation is the process by which a given part of the circulation, in this case the brain, maintains a constant flow of blood over a wide range of blood pressure. This means that the blood flow to the brain is the same if the blood pressure is high or low. This process will only work over a certain range of pressures.

Brain attack: A brain attack is another term for a stroke. Stroke specialists are using this term to communicate the emergency condition, just like a heart attack.

Brain catheterization: Just as a heart catheterization is done for heart attack patients, brain catheterization is increasingly being done for stroke patients. In this procedure, a tiny wire (or catheter) is fed into the brain, where various **endovascular** interventions can then be accomplished.

Brainstem: The brainstem is the lowest portion of the brain, the part that connects the spinal cord with the rest of the brain. Vital bodily functions such as breathing, balance, and many of the cranial nerves have their origin in the brainstem.

Cardiomyopathy: Cardiomyopathy is a disease of the heart that leaves the heart swollen and with a dilated cavity. In this cavity, blood clots can form. Therefore, cardiomyopathy is a risk factor for stroke.

Carotid artery: The carotid arteries are two of the four major arteries that feed the brain. They arise from the **aorta** and its branches. They are a major source of blood to the brain. Blockages can form in the carotid artery, and this situation constitutes a major risk for stroke.

Carotid endarterectomy: Carotid endarterectomy is a surgical procedure that relieves the blockage in the carotid artery. When surgeons perform this procedure, the risk of stroke is markedly lower.

Cerebellum: The cerebellum is in the back portion of the brain and is primarily responsible for balance and coordination.

Cerebral blood flow (CBF): CBF is the blood flow to the brain. This is an important physiological variable. Ultimately, it is the reduced flow of blood to a portion of the brain that causes a stroke.

Cerebral perfusion pressure (CPP): CPP is the pressure that drives blood flow through the brain. The blood pressure must be greater than the pressure that is in the skull, the **intracranial pressure**. In stroke, sometimes the intracranial pressure is elevated, which means the patient's blood pressure must also become elevated to preserve flow to the brain.

Cerebral venous sinus thrombosis (CVST): A CVST is a blood clot that is in the venous (as opposed to arterial) side of the circulation and is a relatively uncommon condition. Clots in these veins can lead to **hemorrhagic stroke**.

Cerebrospinal fluid (CSF): CSF is the clear and colorless fluid that bathes the brain and spinal cord. It is produced in the brain and then reabsorbed. When a doctor does a lumbar puncture to diagnose meningitis or subarachnoid hemorrhage, he is removing a sample of CSF.

Cholesterol: Cholesterol is a fatty substance found in animal fats that is a vital component of normal cells in the body. However, in high levels, it can lead to atherosclerosis and blockages in arteries such as those of the heart and those of the brain.

Circle of Willis: The Circle of Willis is the circular connection of arteries at the base of the brain. This circle connects the **anterior circulation** and the **posterior circulation**. It is a vital portion of anatomy to develop **collateral circulation**.

Coagulopathy: Coagulopathy refers to a problem with blood coagulation. Sometimes, a patient's blood can be too thin, making the patient bleed more easily. Other times, the blood becomes too thick and the patient has a **hypercoagulable state**.

Collateral circulation: Collateral circulation is the body's attempt to provide flow to bypass an obstruction. For example, if the right **vertebral artery** is blocked, blood from other arteries can enter the **Circle of Willis** and feed the arteries that normally would have gotten blood from the blocked vertebral. Think of this like taking a side road around a traffic jam on the road that you had intended to take.

Computed tomography (CT): A CT scan is a powerful kind of x-ray in which x-ray beams are sent in while the receiver spins around the patient. This technique allows doctors to produce incredibly detailed pictures of the brain.

Coumadin: Coumadin (also called warfarin) is a blood thinner, or anticoagulant. It is given to patients with **atrial fibrillation, cardiomyopathy,** and **hypercoagulable states** to prevent strokes.

Cranial nerves: Cranial nerves are bundles of nerve fibers that exit from the **brainstem** and provide control for various bodily functions such as eye movement, sight, hearing, facial expression, tongue movement, and others.

Deep venous thrombosis (DVT): A DVT is a clot in the vein in a body, most commonly in the legs. These blood clots can travel to the heart and sometimes can cross from the right side of the heart to the left side through a **patent foramen ovale** and lead to stroke.

Diabetes: Diabetes is a disease of sugar (or glucose) metabolism. It is an important risk factor for stroke.

Dura: The dura is the outer, tough layer of the **meninges**. Blood can accumulate beneath the dura (a **subdural hematoma**), which is a stroke mimic.

Embolism: An embolism is a clot that has formed in one place and then travels through an artery to another place in the body. An embolism can form in the heart, for example, and then travel to the brain and lead to a stroke.

Endovascular therapy: Endovascular therapy is when a disease state in the body is treated by an intervention that is done from inside of a blood vessel. Heart attacks are routinely treated in this way. Increasingly, patients with subarachnoid hemorrhage and **ischemic stroke** are being treated with endovascular treatments.

Fibrin: Fibrin is a substance in the body that forms a blood clot. It is the target for **fibrinolytic treatments** such as **tissue plasminogen activator**.

Fibrinolytic treatment: Over the past decade or so, doctors are treating patients with fibrinolytic therapy to break up clots in the brain. This treatment has been associated with some controversy, but it is the first treatment that has been shown to improve patient outcomes.

Free radical: These are highly reactive chemicals that are formed in the body. They often contain oxygen and are produced when molecules are oxidized to release products that have unpaired electrons. Free radicals can damage important cellular molecules such as DNA or lipids or other parts of the cell. Substances that reduce free radicals, often called free-radical scavengers, can help reduce this damage.

Frontal lobe of the brain: The frontal lobes are in the front of the brain. They help in many functions of the brain and are largely responsible for thought and planning, coordinating, controlling, and executing behavior. Think of them as being involved with so-called executive functions.

Hemianopsia: Hemianopsia is the word for the symptom in which a patient cannot see to one side or the other. This problem results from destruction (from stroke, tumor, or any other disease) of the portion of the brain that is responsible for vision.

Hemophilia: Hemophilia is a disease of blood coagulation that leads to bleeding and is therefore a risk for **hemorrhagic stroke**.

Hemorrhagic stroke: A hemorrhagic stroke is one in which a blood vessel ruptures and blood escapes into the brain tissue. This can happen with normal blood vessels but more commonly occurs in patients with abnormal vessels such as **aneurysms**, **AVMs**, or the vascular problems associated with **diabetes** or **hypertension**.

Heparin: Like **Coumadin**, heparin is a blood thinner that is used to treat blood clots such as those in **atrial fibrillation**.

Herniation: Herniation is the occasional result of increased **intracranial pressure**. One part of the brain will push (or be pushed by) a wave of pressure against other structures in the skull. If they push against firm, unyielding structures like the **dura**, brain tissue can be destroyed.

Homunculus: The homunculus is the drawing of the distorted human body that represents the way that different parts of the body are supplied by different parts of the brain.

Hypercoagulable state: A hypercoagulable state is one in which the blood clots more easily than normal. This state can lead to clots that form **embolism** that can lead to **ischemic stroke**.

Hypertension: Hypertension, also known as high blood pressure, is a very important risk factor for both **ischemic stroke** and **hemorrhagic stroke**.

Infarction: An infarction means death of tissue. A myocardial infarction is a heart attack. A brain infarction is a stroke.

Internal capsule: The internal capsule is an area of the brain that connects the lower portions of the brain with the higher cortex. It is important because it is an area densely packed with nerve fibers, and strokes in this area sometimes affect large parts of the body.

Intracranial pressure (ICP): Intracranial pressure is the pressure inside of the skull. It is important in many areas of stroke care, both hemorrhagic and ischemic, as well as in the concepts of **cerebral perfusion pressure**. High ICP can lead to brain **herniation**, which can be fatal.

Ischemic penumbra: The area of brain tissue that surrounds the dense core of already dead tissue. This area is ischemic but not yet infarcted, and, therefore, it is still salvageable if treatment can open up the responsible blocked artery.

Ischemic stroke: An ischemic stroke is one in which too little blood flow goes to a given area of the brain, leading to **infarction**.

Lacunar stroke (lacune): Lacunar stroke is a small stroke in an area of brain that is served by a small **penetrating artery** that comes off the **Circle of Willis**. These strokes can be small but sometimes can lead to large neurological deficits.

Lumbar puncture (spinal tap): The lumbar puncture is a diagnostic procedure whereby a doctor places a needle into the **meninges** to collect **cerebrospinal fluid** to diagnose conditions such as meningitis and subarachnoid hemorrhage.

Lumen (of a blood vessel): The lumen is the inside of a blood vessel. A clot forms within the lumen.

Magnetic resonance imaging (MRI): MRI is another way to image the brain and gives doctors even better and more detailed pictures of the brain. In acute stroke, the MRI will sometimes show positive findings within minutes of the event, much sooner than with a **CT scan**.

Mean arterial (blood) pressure (MAP): When you hear a blood pressure of, say, 120 over 80, the upper number is the systolic blood pressure (pressure during the active squeezing of the heart), and the lower number is the diastolic pressure (during the relaxation phase). The MAP is between the two and represents the average pressure over the cardiac cycle.

Medulla: The medulla is the lowest part of the **brainstem** and is the location of important bundles of nerve fibers that descend to and ascend from the spinal cord. Origins of some of the **cranial nerves** are also in the medulla.

Meninges: The meninges are the coverings of the brain and spinal cord. There are three layers: the **dura**, the **arachnoid**, and the **pia**.

Midbrain: A part of the **brainstem**, the midbrain is the site of origin of a number of **cranial nerves**. This part of the brainstem is commonly affected when **herniation** of brain contents occurs.

Neuroplasticity: This refers to the ability of the brain to rearrange neuronal circuits. If one area of the brain is not working properly, the electrical circuits can be rerouted to another area or normally functioning brain tissue.

Neuroprotective drugs: Neuroprotectants are medicines that are meant to protect brain cells after a stroke. Although the concept of neuroprotectants is a good one and one for which there is a lot of experimental evidence, no such drug has been shown to help in actual clinical care. Despite this, numerous studies are ongoing at the present time.

Occipital lobe of the brain: The occipital lobes are in the back part of the brain. They serve as the seat of vision.

Oxygen free radical: See **free radical.**

Paradoxical embolism: A paradoxical embolism is one that starts in the body (usually the leg, as a **deep venous thrombosis**) and then, when the clot starts to move, instead of becoming lodged in the lungs, it crosses over a **patent foramen ovale** and goes to the brain instead, producing an **ischemic stroke.**

Parietal lobe of the brain: The parietal lobe integrates sensory information from different parts of the body, especially those that help with spatial sense and navigation. They help with integrating visual inputs with other sensory information.

Patent foramen ovale (PFO): A PFO is a hole in the upper chambers of the heart that allows for clots that might otherwise travel to the lung, to enter the left side of the heart. These clots then enter the aorta and could go to the brain, in which case they can result in **ischemic stroke.**

Pathophysiology: Pathophysiology refers to the changes that result from various disease states. So the pathophysiology of stroke would be a decrease in blood flow from a portion of the brain attributable to either decreased blood flow (**ischemic stroke**) or bleeding in the head (**hemorrhagic stroke**).

Penetrating artery: A penetrating artery refers to one of a number of small arteries that come off the **Circle of Willis** that supply blood to small, but important areas of the brain such as parts of the uppermost brainstem and middle portions of the cerebrum. Stroke involving these arteries often results in **lacunar stroke.**

Penumbra: See ischemic penumbra.

Pia: This is the innermost and thinnest layer of the **meninges.**

Platelets: Platelets are one of three solid components of blood (the other two are red and white blood cells). Because platelets participate in blood clotting, **anti-platelet medications** are used in patients with **TIA** to prevent a first stroke and in patients who have had strokes to prevent a recurrence.

Pons: The pons is a portion of the brainstem. It lies above the **medulla** and below the **midbrain.** Important **cranial nerves** originate from the pons, which also has many bundles of fibers that run up and down.

Posterior circulation: The posterior circulation of the brain refers to the blood vessels that supply the rear portions of the brain. This is mostly the portion of the brain fed by the two vertebral arteries that arise in the neck and then enter the brain. These arteries and their branches feed the **cerebellum,**

brainstem, and the **occipital lobes**. The posterior circulation is connected to the **anterior circulation** by the **Circle of Willis**.

Procoagulant (drug) therapy: These are drugs given to help the blood clot in situations in which patients have blood that is too thin from **coagulopathy** or from **Coumadin** or **heparin**.

Reperfusion therapy: The underlying **pathophysiology** of ischemic stroke is **infarction** of brain tissue from decreased perfusion to a given area of brain. Reperfusion therapy is any treatment, such as **tissue plasminogen activator** or **endovascular therapy**, that opens up the closed blood vessel.

Retina: The retina is the inside of the eye. It is actually brain tissue and can be affected by a **TIA**. It is also a part of the body that doctors can directly visualize and get a picture of the brain.

Stroke: Otherwise known medically as a brain **infarction**, a stroke is the death of a portion of brain tissue that results from either bleeding or decreased blood flow to a portion of brain.

Subdural hematoma: A subdural hematoma is a collection of blood that lies just inside the **dura**. This can happen from head trauma or sometimes trivial trauma in the setting of a **coagulopathy**.

Telemedicine: Telemedicine refers to the use of broadband television that allows a remote specialist to participate in the care of a patient who might not otherwise have access to such a specialist. The specialist can examine the patient and see the results of imaging studies by remote television.

Thrombosis and thrombus: A thrombus is a clot that forms in the **lumen** of an artery that leads to diminished blood flow and **ischemic stroke**.

Tissue plasminogen activator: This medication can dissolve **fibrin** and is a **fibrinolytic** medication. Its use, although controversial, has been associated with improved patient outcomes.

tPA: See tissue plasminogen activator.

Transient ischemic attack (TIA): A TIA is a very brief episode of brain ischemia that can be caused by all the same things that cause stroke. The correct diagnosis of TIA and treatment of the underlying cause is one important method to prevent strokes.

Triglycerides: Fatty substances in the body that, in high levels, constitute a risk factor for **ischemic stroke**.

Vertebral artery: The two vertebral arteries arise low in the neck and climb into the skull. They supply the blood flow to the **posterior circulation**.

Vertigo: Vertigo is the sense of illusory motion usually described as a sense of spinning. It is a symptom that sometimes will occur with a stroke or TIA but more commonly is seen in problems with the inner ear.

Bibliography

The following is a list of references for readers who want to further research the topic of stroke. Most of the non-website references can also be accessed via the Web; the websites given below were all accessed in September through October 2007. On the websites listed below, one can often find other useful information by navigating within the site and by following links supplied on the site.

American Heart Association. "American Stroke Association" (homepage). http://www.americanheart.org/presenter.jhtml?identifier=4464.

———. "Caring for Someone with Aphasia." http://www.strokeassociation.org/presenter.jhtml?identifier=9063 (website that targets caregivers of patients whose disability includes impaired language function).

———. "Heart and Stroke Encyclopedia." http://www.americanheart.org/presenter.jhtml?identifier=10000056.

———. "Heart Disease and Stroke Statistics—2008 Update." http://www.americanheart.org/presenter.jhtml?identifier=3000090 (some statistics on cardiovascular disease, especially heart disease and stroke).

———. "High Blood Pressure and Stroke." http://www.strokeassociation.org/presenter.jhtml?identifier=9057 (website about high blood pressure and stroke).

———. "How Stroke Affects Behavior: Our Guide to Physical and Emotional Changes." http://www.strokeassociation.org/presenter.jhtml?identifier=9064 (website on the physical and behavioral changes that can follow a stroke).

———. "Know the Facts, Get the Stats." http://www.americanheart.org/presenter.jhtml?identifier=3000996.

————. "Living with Disability after Stroke." http://www.strokeassociation.org/presenter. jhtml?identifier=9061 (website on living with disability after a stroke targeted toward the patient).

————. "Sex after Stroke: Our Guide to Intimacy after Stroke." http://www. strokeassociation.org/presenter.jhtml?identifier=9065 (website that helps patients and their partners with their questions and issue about sexual activity after a stroke).

————. "Stroke: Are You at Risk?" http://www.strokeassociation.org/presenter.jhtml? identifier=9054 (website about risk factors).

————. "There's No Filter for the Truth: Our Guide to Smoking and the Risk of Stroke." http://www.strokeassociation.org/presenter.jhtml?identifier=9059 (website about smoking cigarettes and stroke).

————. "Warning Signs of Stroke: Our Easy-Reading Guide to Emergency Action." http://www.strokeassociation.org/presenter.jhtml?identifier=9058 (website about warning signs of stroke).

Australian Broadcasting Corporation Health & Wellbeing. "Fact File: Stroke." http:// www.abc.net.au/health/library/stories/2002/08/22/1831064.htm (website devoted to some of the historical aspects of stroke).

Caplan LR. "Cerebrovascular Disease: Historical Background with an Eye towards the Future." *Cleveland Journal of Medicine* 71 (January 2004) (a scientific paper on stroke that discusses discoveries over the past few centuries and beyond).

Falcon M, Shoop S. "Basic Instinct May Have Saved Sharon Stone." *USA Today*, October 21, 2001.

MacMullan J. "Bruschi Plans to Play Next Year." *Boston Globe*, September 2, 2005.

————. "Bruschi Will Try to Return." *Boston Globe*, October 15, 2005.

National Institutes of Health. "National Institute of Neurological Disorders and Stroke" (homepage). http://www.ninds.nih.gov.

National Stroke Association (homepage). http://www.stroke.org/site/PageNavigator/ HOME.

Washington University in St. Louis Stroke Center (homepage). http://www. strokecenter.org.

Index

About the Author

JONATHAN A. EDLOW is associate professor of medicine at Harvard Medical School and attending physician at Beth Israel Deaconess Medical Center in Boston. He is the author of *Bullseye: Unraveling the Medical Mystery of Lyme Disease* (2004).